Calculations for Nursing and Healthcare

Diana Coben and
Elizabeth Atere-Roberts

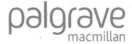

First edition 1996
Reprinted 6 times
Published 2005 by
PALGRAVE MACMILLAN
Houndmills, Basingstoke, Hampshire RG21 6XS and
175 Fifth Avenue, New York, N.Y. 10010
Companies and representatives throughout the world

PALGRAVE MACMILLAN is the global academic imprint of the Palgrave Macmillan division of St. Martin's Press, LLC and of Palgrave Macmillan Ltd. Macmillan® is a registered trademark in the United States, United Kingdom and other countries. Palgrave is a registered trademark in the European Union and other countries.

ISBN-13: 978–1–4039–4078–0
ISBN-10: 1–4039–4078–9

This book is printed on paper suitable for recycling and made from fully managed and sustained forest sources.

A catalogue record for this book is available from the British Library.

10 9 8 7 6 5 4 3 2
15 14 13 12 11 10 09 08 07 06

Printed and bound in China

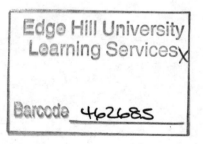

Contents

List of tables and charts

Foreword to the first edition, *Carefree Calculations for Healthcare Students*

When asked to write this foreword, I was struck by the title of the book: '*Carefree* calculations for healthcare students'. For me it embodies the essence of the relationship that should exist between healthcare workers and the mathematical skills that are necessary for them to function efficiently and safely. Healthcare students need to learn to perform the mathematical tasks that they encounter in their everyday life with accuracy and confidence. As members of a 'caring profession' they need to be able to devote that 'care' to their patients, without being distracted by worries associated with the arithmetic they need to do. Healthcare workers need a wide range of skills and abilities at their fingertips, and mathematics – or rather, a very small subset of the mathematical skills taught in the school curriculum – is but one of these. To my mind, it makes little sense automatically to exclude from the profession someone who has all the necessary motivational, academic and empathetic attributes and lacks only a facility in certain areas of arithmetic. On the other hand, one cannot get away from the fact that accurate mathematical calculation can be vital, in the true meaning of that word. Erroneous calculation of drug doses could be fatal. Research undertaken a few years ago (Pirie, 1987) demonstrated that such mathematical deficiency could, however, be remedied during a nurse's training and that what those entering the healthcare profession need, therefore, is a way to assess their mathematical skills to a safe, competent level. 'Care*free*' must not be confused with 'care*less*'.

In today's climate, health workers are faced with ever-expanding responsibility for areas outside their direct sphere of contact with patients. It has become increasingly necessary for them to be able to interpret the data and results reported in medical research and to develop the skills of managing their own budgets. All of this can raise the level of maths anxiety that so many people seem to possess, and come between the nurse and the care owed to the patient. Indeed the more anxious the nurse, the harder it becomes to calculate calmly and accurately. This book addresses this problem head on. Readers are asked to assess their own fears as well as their calculating abilities. They are shown ways to understand how they best learn and then build on their strengths to the point where mathematics no longer causes that low trembling of panic. Individuals are reassured that they are not alone with their worries, but that they cannot shrug off the responsibility for their own learning.

I wish wholeheartedly to endorse the authors' sentiments when they say that healthcare workers owe it to themselves and their patients to be 'competent, confident and comfortable' in all the aspects of mathematics that impinge on their professional lives.

Dr Susan Pirie
September 1995

Foreword to the second edition

Since the first edition of this book was published in 1995, nurses have acquired far greater access to information technology and digital equipment. There has been a rapid proliferation of computers and gadgets both at work and at home, many of which are designed to take the strain off manual methods of measurement and calculation. For example, rather than needing to read off scales such as those on oral thermometers or sphygmomanometers, we are now much more likely to be presented with digital readings from tympanic thermometers or dynamaps. The application of digital technology is greatly advantageous – it enables a far higher degree of accuracy than manual methods did, together with safety and reassurance for the patient. It also saves us time on individual tasks although, paradoxically, time often appears to be proportionally scarcer, as the amount of overall technological support increases!

Diana Coben and Elizabeth Atere-Roberts' revision of their excellent text reminds readers why, despite having gadgets available as never before, the basic maths needed in healthcare has not changed. It is more vital than ever that we are numerate, and vigilant, in interpreting information within a changing clinical environment. Digital readings can be far more precise than most manual readings, but they also have the potential to present results to several decimal places, even if that level of accuracy is not needed. This book will leave you in no doubt of how to tackle the dreaded decimal place. It will help you understand numbers sufficiently to confidently calculate drug doses, interpret readings and charts, recognise normal ranges, manage budgets and oversee duty rotas.

This edition takes into account the impact of all the relevant changes such as the gradual replacement of sphygmomanometers with dynamaps for blood pressure measurement, and the latest assessment tools such as the MUST nutrition tool. It is packed with examples that relate essential maths to current practice, and it acknowledges how nurses actually make calculations and the types of errors they make. A useful feature of the updated edition is the inclusion of many more website addresses for further information.

The authors have retained the reassuring and confidence-building approach that is the joy of the first edition. From the start, they instil a sense of being taken by the hand whilst they help you to develop a positive attitude towards developing maths skills. Triggers of anxiety and stress are confronted and dealt with through building both the coping strategies and the numeric skills that are needed.

This is why the book is so effective; it helps the reader address the whole psychology of their use of maths, as well as the practicalities within an increasingly digital age. This is why the second edition will ensure that nurse readers still emerge as competent, confident, and comfortable as those who were introduced to it in 1995.

Nicky Hayes
Consultant Nurse for Older People

May 2005

Preface to the second edition

This book is the result of a collaboration: it reflects the complementary insights and experience we bring from our respective backgrounds in teaching and research on adult learning of mathematics (Diana Coben) and nursing and healthcare education (Elizabeth Atere-Roberts). We hope that it will be useful to those for whom it was written – nursing and healthcare students and professionals.

We wish to acknowledge the other collaborations which have made essential contributions to the book, especially that with Joan O'Hagan of NIACE (the national organisation for adult learning), with whom the book was conceived. Dr Susan Pirie, formerly of the Mathematics Education Research Centre, University of Oxford, gave generously of her time and insights from her pioneering research in this area at the outset of the project. We have drawn on research on mathematics in nursing and healthcare and on adult learning. Diana Coben's research, with Gillian Thumpston, on adults' mathematics life histories (Coben and Thumpston 1996) informed much of the thinking behind this book, especially Part one, '*Learning and you*'.

This new revised second edition includes much new material throughout, including: non-medical prescribing; the care of older patients; the organisation of nursing and other healthcare work, including staffing and holiday rotas; the use of calculators in the nursing and healthcare context; drug dosage calculations, taking account of new forms of drug packaging; new equipment, such as the replacement of mercury thermometers with new machines measuring the vital signs; and a revised section on demographic profiles drawing on data from the 2001 Census and elsewhere.

We are grateful to staff at Palgrave Macmillan for their vision and commitment to a maths book with a difference, especially Frances Arnold, Kerry Lawrence, Richenda Milton-Thompson and Margaret O'Gorman with respect to the first edition, and to Jon Reed and Lynda Thompson with respect to this second edition.

Our thanks especially to the friends, colleagues and anonymous nursing and healthcare students and professionals who read drafts of the book and whose detailed comments were very helpful indeed. In particular, we are grateful to the following: Ruth Hudson of the Health Visitors' Association; Ena Ertherton of the former West Lambeth Community Care Trust; Dr Sirita Fonseca of the former Wandsworth Community Care Trust; Barbara Jesson of Southwark Primary Care Trust; Sandy Black of the University of the Arts; and the anonymous reviewers – we hope they will recognise improvements in the book as a result of their efforts. Colleagues and friends in Lambeth, Southwark and Lewisham Primary Care Trusts, King's College London and ALM (*Adults Learning Mathematics: A Research Forum*[1]) contributed ideas, helpful criticism and that essential ingredient, enthusiasm. John Ashworth's unfailing support and encouragement throughout have been invaluable.

Any faults or omissions remaining are entirely the responsibility of the authors.

Diana Coben and Elizabeth Atere-Roberts

---

1 *Adults Learning Mathematics: A Research Forum* (ALM) is an international research forum bringing together researchers and practitioners in adult mathematics/numeracy teaching and learning in order to promote the learning of mathematics by adults (www.alm-online.org).

Note to the reader and acknowledgements

The notation used in this book is that of the *British National Formulary* (BNF).

The authors and publishers would like to thank Castlemead Publications for permission to reproduce the boys' growth assessment chart on page 31 and BAPEN for permission to reproduce the MUST chart on page 41. Crown copyright material is reproduced on pages 60–5 with the permission of the Controller of HMSO and the Queen's Printer for Scotland.

Introduction

This book is for you if you are a nurse or healthcare professional or student and you are concerned about your maths.

Our aim is to help you to get to grips with the maths you need to practise safely and effectively.

We start from the premise that many adults' mathematical knowledge and ability to apply that knowledge in different situations is patchy and that we all learn best when what we learn relates directly to our perceived needs and interests.

By the end of this book you should be free to concentrate on caring for patients rather than worrying about your maths. You should know more maths in a nursing and healthcare context, understand it better and have a greater understanding of yourself as a learner. You should have strategies in place to help you if you get stuck and to help you calculate under pressure.

The book is designed for 'open learning'; in other words, you can use it on your own or in a group of friends, colleagues or fellow-students, with or without a teacher. You don't have to read all the parts or do all the tasks – concentrate on the sections that relate to your needs and interests. However, we recommend that you *don't* skip the first part, 'Learning and you'. It should help you to deal with any stress and to manage your time better, since we know from research that it is more difficult to do maths when you're feeling anxious and rushed (Buxton, 1981). It should also help you to get to know yourself better as a learner through exploring your relationship with maths – your maths life history – in order to tackle the maths you need for nursing and healthcare.

Our approach throughout is rooted in research into the use of maths in nursing and healthcare and into adult learning.

Since Susan Pirie's ground-breaking work in the early 1980s (Pirie 1981; 1982) several studies have shown that many nursing and healthcare students and qualified practitioners have difficulty with maths at a fairly basic level (Hek, 1994; Miller, 1993; Dexter & Applegate, 1990; Pirie, 1987). Many also have significant levels of anxiety about mathematics (Fulton & O'Neill, 1989).

At the same time, nurses and other healthcare professionals are having to deal with increasingly complex working environments requiring mathematical ability. For example, nurses nowadays have to cope with complicated drug regimes; research; devolved budgets; new equipment; and issues of accountability to employers, to the public and to their professional organisation. We agree with Hutton (2000), who argues that numeracy must become a priority for nurses.

In organising the book we have drawn on research into adult learning which stresses the importance of 'situated learning' in context (Lave & Wenger, 1991). Situated learning is a holistic model of learning seen as active interaction between the person and their environment: their relationships with other people, their feelings, motivation and values and the tools they use. Alan Schoenfeld, who uses situated learning in his research on mathematics and problem solving, argues that learning to think mathematically means developing both a mathematical point of view and competence with the tools of the trade in order to make mathematical sense of the world (Schoenfeld, 1994). We hope this book will help you to learn in a holistic way, and to think mathematically about your practice.

In Part one we suggest you think about your maths life history. Research into adults' maths life histories has identified the following themes, some of which may chime with your experience:

- The *brick wall* – the point (usually in childhood) at which mathematics stopped making sense; for some people it was long division, for others fractions or algebra, while others never hit the brick wall. For those who did, the impact was often traumatic and long-lasting.
- The *'significant other'* – someone perceived as a major influence on the person's maths life history. The influence might be positive or negative, past or present. Significant others included, for example, a parent who tried to help with maths homework; a teacher who made the person feel stupid; a partner who undermined the person's confidence in their mathematical abilities.
- The *door* – marked 'Mathematics', locked or unlocked, which people have to go through to enter or get on in a chosen line of work or study.
- *Invisible maths* – the mathematics someone can do, but which they may not think of as maths at all, 'just common sense'.

(adapted from Coben & Thumpston, 1996: 288)

In Part two we focus on maths in the nursing and healthcare context, with links to 'Maths refreshers' in Part three. These 'maths refreshers' are designed to refresh your memory, fill any gaps in your knowledge and understanding and build on your experience, using informal methods that you can do in your head as well as using pen and paper or a calculator.

Since the first edition of this book was published in 1996 (Coben & Atere-Roberts, 1996), there have been many changes in the equipment in use in nursing and healthcare and this revised second edition reflects these changes. New technologies make new demands on practitioners' abilities to estimate and exercise their mathematical judgement, while sometimes minimising the need for routine calculation. Indeed, one study found that nurses' mathematical skills were being lost through underuse because of the reduced need for arithmetic calculation, due to the sophisticated technology employed in clinical areas (Cartwright, 1996).

There are several reasons why maths is as important as ever in nursing and healthcare. However sophisticated the technology may be, you need to be able to spot any anomalies and take appropriate action. For example, you need to decide whether a reading on a monitor makes sense in relation to the patient's condition and treatment – perhaps the machine has not been correctly calibrated or is not working properly – that judgement is informed by mathematics, even if you don't do an actual calculation. Also, you need to be able to check your own and your colleagues' calculations and you need not just to be able to estimate and calculate accurately but to know *when* it is appropriate to estimate or do a calculation.

This becomes easier with experience gained in practice, as shown in Meriel Hutton's study of student nurses in a revision programme on nursing mathematics. The students reported that the mathematics they learned only made sense to them through doing it in practice. Accordingly, Hutton recommends that students should be encouraged to maximise their opportunities to practise mathematics in the clinical setting (Hutton 1998a).

One rather surprising side effect of experience is that much of the maths in nursing and healthcare seems to become invisible to experienced practitioners. For example, Hoyles, Noss and Pozzi found mathematics underlying many nursing practices, but unrecognized by nurses themselves. They found that mathematics is closely bound up with contextual factors specific to workplaces and tasks; experienced nurses exercise their judgement through their knowledge of the context as well as their mathematical skills (Noss, Hoyles & Pozzi, 1998). They also noted that workers use equipment of various kinds when making decisions involving mathematics, although they may be unaware of doing so. They conclude that the use of mathematics in the workplace depends on whether the activity is routine or non-routine and on the resources available.

One widely-used resource is the calculator. Hutton investigated student nurses' mathematics and nurses' use of calculators on the ward (Hutton 1998a; 1998b) as did Shockley et al. (1989). Hutton (1998b) found that calculators were used extensively in children's nursing and in high-tech areas of adult nursing. She recommends that nurses working in these areas need both to be able to use calculators accurately and to estimate the correct answer as a checking mechanism; accordingly, both strategies are included in this book.

Our decision to focus on forms of drug packaging and on the organisation of nursing/healthcare work is also informed by research by Hoyles, Noss and Pozzi (2001). They investigated the ways in which expert nurses calculate error-critical drug dosages on the ward, related to the mathematical concepts of ratio and proportion. They found that experienced nurses use a range of correct proportional-reasoning strategies based on the invariant of drug concentration to calculate dosage on the ward, rather than the formula they had been taught in schools of nursing: 'what you want over what you've got, times the amount it comes in'. These calculation strategies are tied to individual drugs in specific quantities and volumes, the way they are packaged, and the ways in which clinical work is organised (Hoyles, Noss & Pozzi, 2001). We've included the drug dosage calculation formula (in Part two), since it's commonly taught and you'll be expected to know it if you don't already, but we've kept our eyes firmly on the ways drug dosages are actually calculated and administered in practice. We've also explained the principle of ratio and proportion (in Part three) to help you understand why the formula works, and we've given you tasks to practise and become familiar with the calculations involved. We have also borne in mind research on different types of medication calculation errors in nursing practice (Bliss-Holtz, 1994).

The problem is that calculation errors can mean real danger for patients and the end of the practitioner's career. We believe that many people who struggle with maths nevertheless have a great deal to offer in nursing and healthcare – *if* they can only overcome their difficulties with maths.

This book is dedicated to liberating that potential.

Part one
Learning and you

▶ Introduction

This chapter aims to help you to get to know yourself better as a learner in order to tackle the maths you need for healthcare.

▶ 1.1   Getting to know yourself as a learner

Start by reflecting on your past and present experiences with maths. One way to do this is by writing your 'maths life history' (see Coben & Thumpston, 1996, for a report on research into adults' maths life histories).

Take some time to think about the following questions in relation to your past and present experiences with maths in any aspect of your life. Note down your thoughts as you go and use your notes as the basis for writing your own maths life history.

Your maths life history
1   How would you describe your feelings about mathematics? In what circumstances do these feelings arise?
2   Describe one thing that you enjoy and one thing that you hate that involve maths.
3   Thinking back over your past life, what events involving maths stand out in your memory?
4   How would you describe your school experiences of maths?
5   In what circumstances do you work out something mathematical . . .
   • in your head?
   • on paper?
   • with a calculator?
   • another way . . . how?

6 When and how do you calculate accurately . . .
  - using whole numbers ?
  - using fractions, including decimal fractions?
7 When and how do you estimate rather than calculate accurately?
8 Describe situations in which you measure each of the following: length; weight; capacity.
9 What activities do you engage in which involve an appreciation of, or the manipulation of, shape and spatial relationships?
10 What effect do you think your experience of maths has had on your opportunities in life?

When you have written your maths life history, put it aside in a safe place; we'll ask you to look back on it later. You don't need to show it to anyone else unless you want to.

▶ 1.2   Developing learning strategies and study skills

Writing your maths life history is designed to get you thinking about the maths in your life in ways you may not have done before. It's a first step towards developing learning strategies and study skills that will stand you in good stead as you progress through this book.

Keeping a maths diary
The next step is to start a 'maths diary' in which to record:

- notes on maths as it arises in a healthcare context
- your thoughts and feelings about the maths that you encounter
- any points of information about maths
- any study tips that you want to remember.

Your maths diary may take any form; most people use either an exercise book or a ring binder, but some prefer a 'proper' diary with the dates already printed. You'll need to allow at least a page a day and to allocate time to writing it up – choose a time that suits you and the pattern of your days.

Keeping a maths diary will make you more aware of the maths in your life: you'll find you notice things that you might previously have missed and you'll become more aware of yourself as a learner in an aspect of your life which you might previously have ignored.

You will find references to your maths diary throughout this book. As with your maths life history, you don't need to show it to anyone else unless you want to.

Talking to colleagues

This may not sound like a learning strategy but it can be very effective. Find a colleague or fellow-student who shares some of your own feelings about maths (preferably someone who has also written his or her maths life history) and talk to each other about the maths in your lives. Ask them to be your 'learning partner' and agree to help each other, working through this book together.

It's important to agree ground rules so that you know what you can expect of each other. Here are some ideas:

- Share strategies for working out maths problems – remember there's nearly always more than one way of doing a mathematical operation and the 'right' way is the way that works – it's also a good idea to double-check your answer using a different method.
- Talk through your feelings about maths – if something doesn't feel right to you, even if you know it gives the correct answer, talk it over with your partner and you may find that a different way of looking at the problem helps you to see it more clearly.
- Talk over the situations you come across that involve maths, especially those which involve doing maths under pressure, and share strategies for remaining calm and doing the maths.

Getting to know your number-crunching skills

In this section you are going to look at how you tackle a range of calculations, for example:

- What kinds of number-crunching strategies do you use?
- What do you do when things go wrong?

Calculations vary in terms of how difficult they are and different people prefer different ways of tackling them. For all methods you have to do some thinking first, but when you start doing the number-crunching you have a choice: you can do the calculations on paper or in your head, or you can use a calculator. Whichever method you choose, it's a good idea to use a different method to check your result.

Activities – Learning and you

Task 1 Which number-crunching method do you prefer?

Spend about 20 minutes doing this exercise with your learning partner.

The aim of the exercise is for you to observe which number-crunching method you're inclined to use in different situations.

You don't have to do the actual calculations at this stage; just observe your reactions and which method you're inclined to favour. Sometimes you may need to start the problem so that you can decide which number-crunching method you'd prefer to use; but don't try to finish them.

Read each problem, and **record** on Table 1 which number-crunching method (with a calculator, in your head, or on paper) you prefer to use. Use the third column in the table to write down your reaction to the problem, for example:

- *easy*
- *made me panic*
- *this kind of problem always gives me trouble.*

Spend about five minutes on this. Then discuss your observations with your learning partner.

Table 1 *Which number-crunching method do you prefer?*

Problem	Your method	Comments
1 A 1.8m-tall man weighed 100kg on admission to hospital. He was put on a special diet and is losing weight at a rate of 3kg each week. How long will it take him to reach a target weight in the range 58–83kg?	*(handwritten working)* 0̶1̶0̶0̶ 83 − ——— 17 5.33 3)17 15 020 18 20	
2 A baby's birth weight is 4kg. She loses and then regains 10% of her birth weight in her first two weeks of life. How low does her weight go during the first two weeks?	*(handwritten)* 3.6Kg	

○ ○ ▷

Problem	Your method	Comments
3 A drug dose of 62.5mg is available as 25mg in 1ml. What is the dose in millilitres? *2.5ml*	$\overset{\cdot}{2} = 50$ $2.5ml = 62.5$	
4 Convert 0.075mg to micrograms.		

Task 2   Analysing errors

In this section we ask you to complete some calculations and to think about possible sources of error.

Look back at the problems in Task 1, and this time do the calculations. Then fill in the "how confident . . ." column in Table 2. Check your answers with ours (at the back of the book) and record in the third column whether you got them right or wrong.

Table 2   *Analysing errors*

	How confident I feel	Whether I was right or wrong
1		
2		
3		
4		

If you were confident about all of them, and you got them all right, try this exercise with another set of calculations drawn from elsewhere in the book.

If you were not very confident, or if you got some wrong, what do you think might have gone wrong?

○ ○ ▷

You might have:

- misread the numbers in the question
- made an arithmetic slip, e.g., $3.0 + 4.5 = 7$
- used the wrong formula
- used the right formula but put in the wrong numbers
- multiplied or divided the wrong numbers.

In your maths diary, note down the kinds of error you made.

Task 3   How do you react to any errors?

Now think about your reactions if you got some answers wrong.

What were you inclined to do or think?

Tick the boxes below which apply to you:

Table 3   *How do you react to any errors?*

Forget my first attempt and start again	
Forget the whole problem and do something else	
Try to do the same operation but with easier numbers	
Go back to the problem to read it more carefully	
Check my written work to look for mistakes	
Wish I'd written something down so that I could check it	
Ask somebody else to look at my work and check it for me	
Take a break to clear my head	
Look up the formula somewhere	
Blame the calculator	
It doesn't surprise me that I got it wrong	
There must be a mistake in the book	

Now you know what you tend to do when you get stuck, read through the other options again and consider using some of them as well.

○ ○ ▷

Task 4   Developing a feel for what's likely

Another important aspect of analysing errors is developing a feel for what's likely and spotting the unlikely in a healthcare context.

Which of the following is unlikely?

Table 4   *Developing a feel for what's likely*

Injecting 50ml of digoxin

Giving a patient 50ml of medicine orally

A prescription of phenobarbitone 180mg orally at night

Giving 0.02ml as an oral dose

An application of ichthammol ointment 3 times daily

Giving a child 6 tablets in one dose

Look again at the 'unlikely' options in Table 4. What do you think might have gone wrong in each case?

- A mistake in the calculation?
- The prescribing doctor has made a mistake?
- The dosage has been misread or misheard?
- The stock solution is mislabelled?

As you see, not all errors involve calculation.

Cultivate an awareness of different types of error and you will be able to spot errors more easily and take appropriate action.

Use a *British National Formulary* (*BNF*) to check the prescription whenever you feel unsure.

▶ **1.3   Time and stress management**

Even the most meticulously careful person is more likely to make a mistake when working under pressure – something which healthcare professionals have to do for much of the time. It's important, therefore, to learn how to calculate and estimate under pressure.

This section is designed to help you to manage your time and stress levels to enable you to calculate and estimate under pressure.

Time management

Good management of time means making the best use of whatever time is available. Nurses and other healthcare professionals need to manage their time as efficiently as possible in order to cope with the increasing complexity and volume of work involved in providing an efficient healthcare service.

The key to effective time management is *planning and prioritising in relation to context* – i.e. the type of healthcare setting (for example, long-stay continuing care or acute care, hospital or community-based) and the healthcare team of which you are a part.

Planning and prioritising effectively ensures that while everything may not be done in the time available, that which has been identified as high priority by the healthcare team is done; the rest is kept on the agenda for future action.

But what counts as high priority? Time spent with patients and their relatives/carers assessing the patients' needs and planning, delivering and evaluating their care is important, but is it more important than ensuring that medication is given correctly? Time must also be allocated to those aspects of healthcare which underpin patient care, such as ensuring that enough staff are available to maintain the quality of the service.

Your priorities and the scope of your planning will depend to some extent on the nature of your particular responsibilities as a member of the healthcare team.

You must also be able to distinguish between that which is *important* and that which is *urgent* – these are not always the same thing. For example, it may be urgent that a sample of a patient's blood is sent for testing before the laboratory closes, while it may be important to spend time with a dying patient. Priorities often conflict and you will need to make a professional judgement in each instance. In the above situation, you would need to consider whether a colleague could take the blood sample, or alternatively, spend time with the dying patient. If there is no one else available, you would need to weigh up the amount of time needed to take the sample, against the likelihood of the patient dying in the meantime. You would also need to consider the 'opportunity cost' (that which would be lost) if one or other is not done. Ask yourself 'What is the worst that could happen in this situation?'

In his book *Effective Time Management*, John Adair sets out 'Ten Steps Towards Better Time Management' (Adair, 1988: 151):

• Develop a personal sense of time

- Identify long-term goals
- Make middle-term plans
- Plan the day
- Make best use of your time
- Organise office work
- Manage meetings
- Delegate effectively
- Make use of committed time
- Manage your health.

Tick off the items on the list which apply to you – for instance, you may not have anyone to whom you can delegate work, or you may not be involved in meetings on a regular basis, but you *can* develop a personal sense of time, for example by keeping a record of your use of time over a period of a week in your maths diary and then reviewing your use of time. Write down each point which applies to you in your maths diary.

Now see if any of the items you have *not* ticked can be adapted to suit your circumstances. For example, you may not do any 'office work' as such, but perhaps you could organise your notes so as to make it easier to find topics and so make the best use of your time for study. Add the adapted items to your list.

Are there any other items which you think should be added? If so, add these to the list – but *don't* make the list too long.

Look again at your list. Make a note beside each point of the circumstances in which it comes into play. For example, 'plan the day' could be something you choose to do each morning in the bathroom or on the bus, or you could set aside a few minutes at the end of each day to plan the next day.

Try managing your time on this basis for a week and then review your progress in your maths diary, noting down and changing anything that didn't work out. Review your progress again after one month.

If you're successful in improving your management of time, you should find you have more time to do the things you enjoy and that you enjoy life more now that you are able to pace yourself – you should notice a reduction in the amount of stress in your life. The next section looks at stress management.

Stress management

Caring for people who are ill, bereaved or having problems can be very stressful, so does this mean that the health of all nurses and other health-care professionals is at risk? The answer is 'yes' and 'no'. Stress is not a disease, and can lead to improved performance when sustained for short periods. Stress becomes a problem and can lead to illness when it is repeated and prolonged. Stress is inherent in healthcare: it can't be avoided altogether but it can be minimised and you can learn to manage stress productively.

People experience and deal with the effects of stress in different ways, physically, emotionally and socially, and it is known that people with certain personality types suffer more from the effects of stress than others. It is also often easier to see the effects of stress on others and overlook the effects on yourself.

Becoming aware of the stress in your life is the key to developing coping mechanisms which enable you to meet the demands of your work – mathematically and otherwise – and enjoy a balance between work and the rest of your life.

But self-awareness is only part of the picture. It is part of a manager's responsibility to reduce unnecessary stress among staff. Unfortunately signs of stress are sometimes seen by managers as indications of failure and consequently staff may be reluctant to seek help.

If you feel that the level of stress in your life is too high and you don't feel able to talk to your manager, talk to your learning partner, or to your partner or a close friend. Often the relief of talking to someone is enough to put the problem into perspective. If not, then you may need to seek professional help from a counsellor.

Meanwhile, try doing a *stress review*.

First, jot down in your maths diary three things which have caused you stress recently. These might include, for example: a row with a colleague; the death of a patient; missing an important study deadline.

Now jot down what you could have done to alleviate the stress you felt in each instance – could you have avoided the problem altogether – for example, by organising your time better so that you didn't miss the study deadline? Could you have minimised the damage, for example by talking over the problem that led to the row with your colleague with her after you'd both calmed down? Was there anything you could or should have done differently in the case of the patient who died? If not, then allow yourself to grieve; it's important to balance professional detachment with compassion and to accept that there are some things that you cannot change.

In each case you can learn from your experience by reflecting on it in order to improve your future performance – and in so doing you will reduce stress.

Repeat your stress review after one week and one month. In the meantime: try to improve your general health through improved diet and exercise; develop ways of relaxing; make time for your nearest and dearest and for yourself. Look again at the section on *time management* – working under constant time pressure is very stressful and if you can improve your management of time you'll find that other things fall into place. Remember that stress in moderation can 'tone you up' – it's too much stress that does damage.

▶ 1.4   Calculating and estimating under pressure

Once you've done your best to alleviate the ill effects of excessive stress and improved your management of time, you can look at ways of calculating and estimating under pressure.

The key here is to start from where you are and develop your strengths in order to minimise any weaknesses.

Start from where you are
First, do a *maths stress review*, similar to your general *stress review* (see above) but focusing particularly on the maths in your life. You might find it helpful to look back at your *maths life history* at this point.

Jot down three things involving maths which have caused you stress recently. These might include, for example: calculating the dosage of a drug with which you are unfamiliar; having to complete a set of calculations in a hurry while someone waits for the results; making a presentation to a group of your colleagues or fellow-students on the basis of some research you have done which involves maths.

Now jot down what you could have done to alleviate the stress you felt in each instance – look at how you tackled the problem and what aids were available to you. In the case of the drug calculation, did you try to do it in your head, on paper or with a calculator? Why did you choose to do it that way? In retrospect, could you have done it better using another method? Were you in too much of a hurry – could you have tackled the calculation if you'd given yourself more time to think? Were you trying to calculate in an unsuitable environment (with distractions, a high level of noise etc.)? Were you tired or tense? If so, look back at the sections on time and stress management and see if you could improve matters. Discuss the problem with your learning partner – what does she or he do in a similar situation?

What if you are unsure of the maths involved *whichever* method you chose in this instance and whatever the circumstances? If so, work through section *2.6 Giving medication* (p. 45).

Develop your strengths

What are your strengths in relation to the maths in your life? The first step towards developing your strengths is to identify them. Look back at your maths life history. If you find it difficult to identify any strengths, sit down with your learning partner and share ideas – it's often easier to see someone else's strong points than your own.

Perhaps you are good at working methodically through problems, or at remembering techniques for problem solving. Perhaps you can see a solution to a problem even if you're not always sure how you got there. You may be good at estimating, or mental arithmetic.

Once you've identified your strengths, make a note of them in your maths diary for future reference. Think of circumstances in which they are particularly useful and of ways in which you can build on them. For example, if you are methodical you probably have considerable patience and good attention to detail, qualities which come into their own in many of the routine tasks required in healthcare. A good memory is very useful; if you can harness your memory to a good understanding of maths so that you use the techniques stored in your memory appropriately, you will go far.

If you have a good intuitive grasp of maths but are less secure on the technical details, learn to value your insights. If you can see what the answer to a problem is but don't know the right method, work backwards – try a few ways of working it out until you find a way that suits the case in point and then try the same method on a similar problem. Remember that there is usually more than one way of solving a maths problem – if the one you try works for several different problems, it's probably OK. If the numbers concerned are awkward, try substituting easier numbers – this may help you to identify an appropriate method. If you're still not sure, look for a similar problem in this book or check with someone whose knowledge and experience you respect.

Many people assume that estimating is a weakness rather than a strength, forgetting that in many situations accurate calculation is not necessary. The important thing is to know when accuracy is required and when estimating is more appropriate. This is partly a matter of common sense and partly of experience – *never* estimate an intravenous (IV) drug dosage, for example, but it is perfectly safe to estimate a patient's fluid loss through perspiration on a fluid balance chart.

If you are good at mental arithmetic, rejoice in the amount you'll save on biros and calculator batteries! This is a really useful skill which will stand you in good stead in many aspects of the maths in healthcare.

Make the most of your strengths. Start thinking of yourself as someone who *can* do maths, rather than as someone who finds maths difficult. Difficult maths is just the maths you can't do – yet!

Minimise any weaknesses

As with your strengths, the first thing to do is to become aware of your weaknesses. Look back at your maths life history. Discuss your weaknesses with your learning partner. Make a list of them in your maths diary and next to each one write down what you can do to overcome it or compensate for it.

For example, if your memory is poor, you probably already make notes or have other techniques for reminding yourself of what you're doing. What helps you to remember things? How could you improve your memory and improve your techniques for remembering things?

If you are careless, prone to making arithmetic slips, train yourself to 'edit' your maths – take your time and *always* check your calculations (you may need to put the calculation aside for a while and come back to it before you notice a mistake).

If you find it difficult to know where to start with a maths problem, take a deep breath, remember your strengths and try to understand what the problem actually entails. This may sound obvious, but people are often unable to 'see through to the maths' in a problem because they're trying – and failing – to remember what they did when they came across a similar problem in the past, or to remember how they were taught to tackle maths problems at school. Either of these approaches might work, but they might also stop you seeing the problem in the light of your *present* knowledge and experience.

The best way to minimise any weaknesses in relation to the maths in your life is by becoming aware of them, seeing them as part of the picture, not the whole thing, and overcoming or compensating for them wherever possible.

It usually helps to discuss the problem with someone – ideally your learning partner – and to write it out in your maths diary as clearly as possible, together with a commentary on what it is you find off-putting about it and your thoughts on how to tackle it.

Some people find maths so frightening that they feel totally unable to face it. If you recognise yourself in this description – don't despair. This book has been written with your needs in mind and there are other books designed to help with maths (see, for example, Coben & Black, 2005) and with maths anxiety (see Zaslavsky, 1994).

Maths is an important aspect of healthcare. As the author of a critical review of the literature on competence in practice-based calculation in nursing education puts it:

We need to develop a broader conception of 'competence' that values the ability to use number skills in creatively interpreting clinical situations, and which incorporates the idea that confidence and competence in number will be clinically useful and professionally valuable. (Sabin, 2001: 39)

We agree: as a nurse or healthcare professional, you need to be

- *competent*
- *confident* and
- *comfortable*

with the maths in your life.

These *three C's* spell success in calculations for nursing and healthcare.

Part two

Calculations in the nursing and healthcare context

▶ Introduction

This part of the book is designed to introduce you to the maths involved in some aspects of nursing and healthcare delivery.

We have focused on topics which are fundamental to all healthcare and now want to look at the maths involved *in context*. Our aim is to cover a range of contexts and particularly to address the needs of those who are just beginning their training. We have therefore included basic healthcare procedures such as monitoring vital signs and explanations of common medical terms.

Use your maths diary to note down the maths you encounter in various healthcare settings. Look for links between topics and situations where the same mathematical operation is used in several different contexts.

Make notes on your feelings about the maths you encounter, the circumstances in which you encountered it and how you coped. What strategies did you use? Did you manage to solve the problem? What previous knowledge and experience did you draw on to solve the problem? Can you identify other situations where you have used the same mathematical operations?

Talk through your feelings and experiences with your learning partner.

The British National Formulary (BNF) website at http://bnf.org/bnf/extra/current/noframes/450016.htm includes calculators for some of the topics covered in this chapter, such as Body Mass Index and Body Surface Area, and others.

▶ 2.1   Monitoring vital signs

Accurate monitoring of the *vital signs: temperature, pulse, respiration* and *blood pressure* is an important nursing procedure.

On admission to hospital patients usually have their temperature, pulse, respiration and blood pressure taken and recorded on a chart such as the *vital signs* chart (see p. 22). This acts as a baseline and will provide you with useful data to work from.

Temperature

Body temperature is the balance between the heat produced and acquired by the body.

Temperature is measured in degrees *Celsius* (also called Centigrade), written °C.

 Connections

Previously the Fahrenheit scale was used. It should not be necessary to convert from Fahrenheit to Celsius or vice versa – it's better to think in Celsius – but if you have to, turn to *3.8 Conversions* (p. 99).

The Celsius scale has 100 degrees (°) between freezing point (0°C) and boiling point (100°C) of water.

Normal room temperature is around 20°C.[1]

Normal body temperature

Normal body temperature varies between people, and even in the same individual it varies depending on age, activity and time of day (for example, temperature is usually higher in the evening) and whether a woman is ovulating or having her menstrual period.

Temperature also varies depending on where it is taken: average normal body temperature, taken orally (in the mouth) or *per axilla* (in the armpit), is 36.7°C–37.2°C; taken rectally or in the ear (tympanic membrane), normal temperature is 37.4°C.

Rectal or ear temperature is 0.3°C to 0.6°C higher than oral temperature. Armpit temperature is 0.3°C to 0.6°C lower than oral temperature.

A child's temperature can vary between 36°C and 37°C.

Infants' and children's body temperature varies daily according to age as follows:

---

1 See Health Guide A-Z for further information on body temperature. (http://my.webmd.com/ hw/health_guide_atoz/hw198785.asp).

- Under 6 months, the daily variation is small.
- From 6 months to 2 years, the daily variation is about 1 degree.
- Daily variations gradually increase to 2 degrees per day by the age of 6.

You need to know what normal body temperature is in order to tell when a patient's temperature is abnormally low or high.

 Connections

In 36.7° the . is the decimal point. In other words, normal body temperature varies from 36 degrees and seven-tenths of a degree Celsius to 37 degrees and two-tenths of a degree Celsius. The number immediately to the left of the decimal point is whole degrees, the figure immediately to the right (the 'first decimal place') is tenths of a degree Celsius.

If you are unsure about decimals turn to *3.3 Decimals and fractions* (p. 79).

You will come across patients who develop a high temperature (*pyrexia*, above 37.5°C, and *hyperpyrexia*, above 39°C).

You will also come across patients, particularly older people and those exposed to cold, whose temperatures are very low (*hypothermia*, below 35°C).

In these life-threatening situations you will need to take prompt action to bring the temperature up or down gradually as necessary.

The speed with which recordings can be obtained and the risk posed by the use of mercury thermometers has led to a switch from these devices to electronic versions.

Mercury thermometers are now used less often; they have been replaced by electronic devices, including tympanic thermometers. These measure the temperature of the tympanic membrane by inserting a probe in the ear canal. The probe at the end of the hand-held device records the temperature and displays the reading on a digital screen. Although quick and easy to use, to ensure accurate measurement staff should be given training in the correct use of these devices based on the manufacturers' instructions.

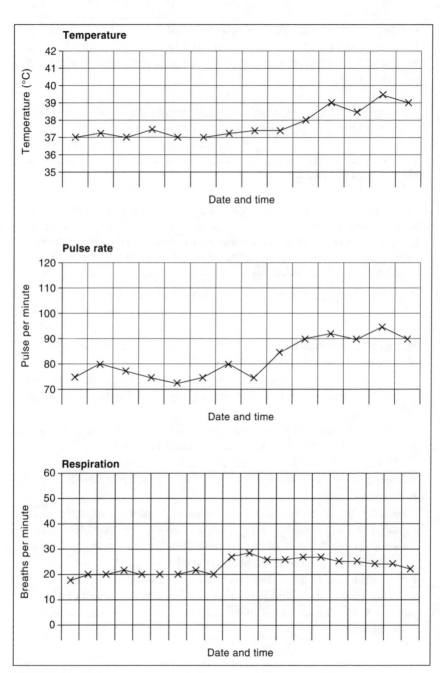

Vital signs charts

Practice tip

Always use a clean, disposable probe cover for each patient to avoid the risk of cross-infection.

Mercury thermometers
On a clinical thermometer, each degree is divided into tenths in order to allow fine distinctions in temperature to be read.

Various clinical thermometers with different scales are used in medicine.

A thermometer with a scale ranging from 25°C to 40°C (a low-grade thermometer) is used to measure the temperature of patients who are *hypothermic*.

A thermometer with a scale ranging from 35°C to 43°C is used to measure the temperature of patients who are *pyrexic* or *hyperpyrexic*.

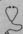

Practice tip

Always shake the thermometer so that the mercury falls to the lowest point on the scale and read and record the temperature carefully – accuracy is very important.

The pulse
The *pulse* is a pressure wave of blood caused by the alternating expansion and recoil of elastic arteries during each cardiac cycle.

The pulse rate is measured in *beats per minute*.

Pulse rate should always be counted for a full minute and not for 15 or 30 seconds. The reason for this is that you could miss vital findings in the omitted 45 or 30 seconds: you would be at risk of making a judgement on your findings from the first 15 or 30 seconds when this might not be the true picture if you had counted for a full minute.

The normal pulse rate for an adult at rest is 60–80 beats per minute.

The normal pulse rate for an infant under one year old at rest is 80–120 beats per minute.

Pulse sites
Several sites in the body may be used for palpating the pulse. The most

common site is the radial artery at the wrist. Other sites are temporal, carotid, brachial, femoral, popliteal and dorsalis pedis arteries.

When you palpate and count the pulse you are doing three main things:

- feeling for the rate (beats per minute)
- feeling for the rhythm (regular or not?)
- feeling for the strength (weak or strong?).

You will come across patients with an abnormally fast pulse rate (*tachycardia* – over 100 beats per minute in adults), and patients with slower heart rate (*bradycardia* – less than 60 beats per minute)

Respiration

The function of the respiratory system is to supply the body with *oxygen* and to remove *carbon dioxide*.

Respiration is measured in *breaths per minute*. The normal respiration rate at rest is approximately 16 to 20 breaths per minute in adults – faster in children and infants.

Respiration involves inspiration and expiration. In inspiration, air moves into the lungs and in expiration, air moves out of the lungs.

As with the pulse, the respiration rate must be taken for a full minute. The patient should not be aware of what you are doing as this might alter the rate.

Some nurses tend to attach less importance to the respiration rate, but this recording is just as important as the other vital signs. In some cases it may be the first sign that something is wrong – for example, if a patient has a chest infection, you may observe that breathing is rapid, laboured or noisy, which would lead you to take the patient's temperature or to send a sputum specimen to the laboratory to confirm the diagnosis.

Blood pressure

Blood pressure is the pressure exerted laterally on the walls of the main arteries by the blood.

Blood pressure is measured in *millimetres of mercury (mmHg)* and expressed as the juxtaposition of systolic pressure and diastolic pressure, for example, '130 over 70 millimetres of mercury', written as '130/70mmHg'.

But what does this mean?

The *systolic* pressure is a measure of the maximum pressure of the blood against the wall of the blood vessel following ventricular contraction.

The *diastolic* pressure is a measure of the minimum pressure of the blood against the wall of the blood vessel following the closure of the aortic valve.

In the case of a patient with blood pressure of 130/70mmHg, the pumping action of the circulatory system is sufficient to support a column of mercury 130 millimetres high.

 Connections

A millimetre (mm) is one-thousandth of a metre (m).
If you are unsure about the metric system, see *3.6 The metric (SI) system* (p. 94).

The normal systolic blood pressure in a healthy young adult is less than 140mmHg. The normal diastolic pressure is less than 90mmHg. Blood pressure between 140–159 (systolic) or 90–99 (diastolic) is mild high blood pressure; blood pressure above 160 (systolic) or above 100 (diastolic) is high blood pressure (BHS 2005).

So a reading of 130/70mmHg means that the maximum pressure of the blood against the wall of the blood vessel following ventricular contraction is 130, and the minimum pressure of the blood against the wall of the blood vessel following the closure of the aortic valve is 70.

What happens when a patient's blood pressure falls outside the normal range?

When the systolic pressure of an adult falls below 100mmHg, the condition is called *hypotension*.

When there is a sustained elevation of the blood pressure of over 160/95mmHg, the condition is called *hypertension*.[2]

The difference between the systolic and diastolic blood pressure is known as the *pulse pressure*.

For example, if systolic pressure is 120mmHg and diastolic pressure is 70mmHg, pulse pressure is 50mmHg because:

$$120 - 70 = 50mmHg$$

---

2 See the British Hypertension Society Guidelines, in *Journal of Human Hypertension* 18 (2004), 139–85 (www.nature.com/jhh).

Dynamap Automated Blood Pressure Sphygmomanometer
Blood pressure is now commonly measured electronically, rather than by mercury sphygmomanometers, in devices which also measure the other vital signs, called Dynamap automated blood pressure sphygmomanometers.

Although no calculation is required for these devices, you need to be aware of the normal range of these recordings in order to interpret the numbers displayed correctly and to make effective clinical judgements.

Practice tip

These devices need to be properly maintained and regularly calibrated.

Activities – Working with the vital signs

Task 1

You are expecting a patient to be admitted with possible hypothermia. In what range would you expect the patient's temperature to be?

Task 2

A patient's blood pressure is 140/90mmHg. What is the patient's pulse pressure?

Task 3

A patient is admitted one evening with an oral temperature of 38°C. Overnight her temperature rises to 41°C. By how much has the temperature risen? Is this a significant rise and, if so, why?

Task 4

A woman is admitted with a severe chest infection. Her respiration rate is 30 breaths per minute. Approximately how much is this above the normal respiration rate?

Task 5

An elderly man is found unconscious on the floor of his flat. His pulse is very faint and you count 45 beats per minute. Approximately how much is this below the normal pulse rate?

▶ 2.2   Measuring weight and height

Body weight is considered in relation to the patient's height.

Some patients are weighed on admission to hospital; in particular, a patient being prepared for surgery will be weighed in order to assess the dosage of anaesthetics required. Some patients will continue to be weighed on a regular basis throughout their stay in hospital. Similarly, in the community, a patient's weight may be monitored regularly.

The patient's weight at the outset of treatment acts as a baseline which may be used, for example, to measure the effectiveness of prescribed drugs or to determine whether a patient on a special diet or treatment is losing or gaining weight and to monitor the retention and output of bodily fluids.

In the metric system (also called the 'SI system', short for *Système International d'Unités* or International System of Units) body weight is measured in *kilograms (kg)*, also known as *kilos*. Height is measured in *metres (m)*, or metres and *centimetres (cm)*.

For example, a woman who measures 1.83m (you'd say 'one metre eighty-three' or 'one metre eighty-three centimetres' or 'one point eight three metres') might weigh 57.15kg (you'd say 'fifty-seven point one five kilos').

Practice tip

When assessing a patient's height:

- Set up a wall chart with 1m and 2m clearly marked.
- Make a mental comparison of the patient with the markings on the chart before you take an accurate measurement.
- This will help you to estimate height and to spot any major errors.

You need to be familiar with kilograms, metres and centimetres in order to measure and record a patient's weight and height accurately. You also need to be able to judge whether a person is overweight or underweight for their height.

 Connections

There's more information about this in *3.6 The metric (SI) system* (p. 94).

If you can't measure an adult patient's height accurately for some reason, for example, if the patient is bedbound and frail, then you can estimate their height by measuring between the point of the elbow and the prominent bone of the wrist and then reading off an estimated height from the chart on the opposite page.

Weight

Start with what you know: a bag of granulated sugar weighs 1 kilogram; most airlines operate a weight limit for a passenger's baggage of 22 kilograms. You may know your own weight in kilos; if not, weigh yourself and this time read the kilogram scale rather than the scale showing stones and pounds (most bathroom scales show both kilograms and stones and pounds). For example, if you weigh 9 stone, you will find that is 57 kilograms (57kg). Record your metric weight in your maths diary. Most medical scales show weight in more detail than domestic bathroom scales, which usually just show whole kilograms and not parts of a kilogram, giving a reading to the nearest kilogram.

Suppose you weigh a child who weighs 26.5kg, what does the '.5' mean?

The 26 (to the left of the decimal point) means 26 whole kilograms.

The .5 (the figure 5 immediately to the right of the decimal point) means five-tenths of a kilogram, which is the same as half a kilogram. So the .5 means 500 grams because there are 1000 grams in one kilogram.

 Connections

See the section on decimals in *3.3 Decimals and fractions* (p. 79).

Accuracy is very important, particularly when weighing babies and young children or anyone undergoing surgery, so, as with any other machinery, weighing scales need to be checked and serviced regularly. The scale should be calibrated to ensure that the readings given are correct.

This weight chart shows an adult's weight recorded daily over a two-week period.

Estimation of height chart

Height (m)														
Men <65 years	1.94	1.93	1.91	1.89	1.87	1.85	1.84	1.82	1.80	1.78	1.76	1.75	1.73	1.71
Men >65 years	1.87	1.86	1.84	1.82	1.81	1.79	1.78	1.76	1.75	1.73	1.71	1.70	1.68	1.67
Ulna length (cm)	32.0	31.5	31.0	30.5	30.0	29.5	29.0	28.5	28.0	27.5	27.0	26.5	26.0	25.5

Height (m)														
Women <65 years	1.84	1.83	1.81	1.80	1.79	1.77	1.76	1.75	1.73	1.72	1.70	1.69	1.68	1.66
Women >65 years	1.84	1.83	1.81	1.79	1.78	1.76	1.75	1.73	1.71	1.70	1.68	1.66	1.65	1.63

Height (m)														
Men <65 years	1.69	1.67	1.66	1.64	1.62	1.60	1.58	1.57	1.55	1.53	1.51	1.49	1.48	1.46
Men >65 years	1.65	1.63	1.62	1.60	1.59	1.57	1.56	1.54	1.52	1.51	1.49	1.48	1.46	1.45
Ulna length (cm)	25.0	24.5	24.0	23.5	23.0	22.5	22.0	21.5	21.0	20.5	20.0	19.5	19.0	18.5

Height (m)														
Women <65 years	1.65	1.63	1.62	1.61	1.59	1.58	1.56	1.55	1.54	1.52	1.51	1.50	1.48	1.47
women >65 years	1.61	1.60	1.58	1.56	1.55	1.53	1.52	1.50	1.48	1.47	1.45	1.44	1.42	1.40

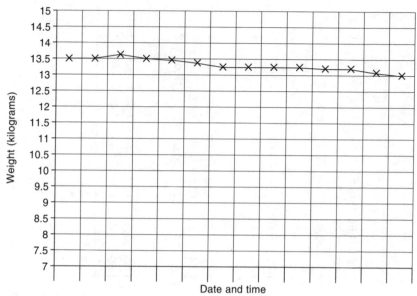

Record of weight chart

Centile chart

The weights of babies and children are recorded on a centile (or percentile) chart. A centile chart allows for adjustment in the recording of a baby's weight according to its date of birth and gestational age. The centile is a relative position, allowing the baby's weight to be judged in relation to what would be expected for a baby of that age, size and gender. In order to establish the values for a centile chart, a group of children of the same age is weighed. For example, 50% (or 50 out of every 100) of baby boys aged 6 weeks, born at term, would be expected to weigh between 4.4kg and 5.1kg, 25% (or 25 out of every 100) would be expected to weigh more than this and 25% would be expected to weigh less (for an example of a centile chart, see the *Boys' Growth Assessment Chart* on p. 31).

Weight in relation to anaesthesia

The patient's weight is also used to assess the amount of anaesthesia to be given – another reason why it is important that patients' weights are accurately recorded. The amount of anaesthesia required varies with individuals; for example, someone who is tall and heavily built requires more than a frail, slight, older person.

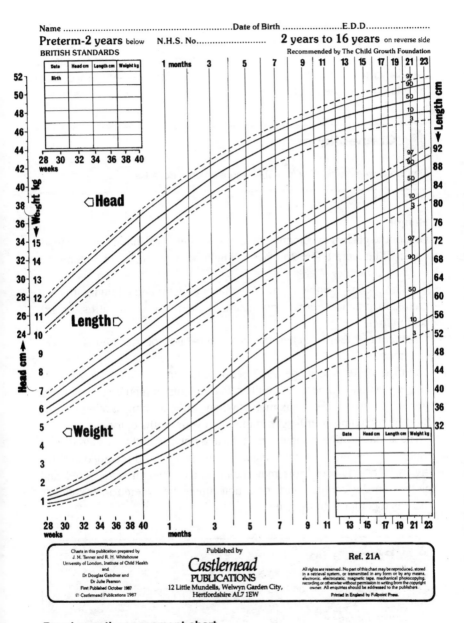

Name ....Date of Birth ......................E.D.D......................

Preterm-2 years below   N.H.S. No.........................   **2 years to 16 years** on reverse side

BRITISH STANDARDS   Recommended by The Child Growth Foundation

Charts in this publication prepared by
J. M. Tanner and R. H. Whitehouse
University of London, Institute of Child Health
and
Dr Douglas Gairdner and
Dr Julie Pearson
First Published October 1987
© Castlemead Publications 1987

Published by

Castlemead
PUBLICATIONS
12 Little Mundells, Welwyn Garden City,
Hertfordshire AL7 1EW

Ref. 21A

All rights are reserved. No part of this chart may be reproduced, stored
in a retrieval system, or transmitted in any form or by any means,
electronic, electrostatic, magnetic tape, mechanical photocopying,
recording or otherwise without permission in writing from the copyright
owner. All enquiries should be addressed to the publishers.

Printed in England by Fullpoint Press.

Boys' growth assessment chart
Reproduced with permission from Castlemead Publications

Weight in relation to drug dosages
Some drug dosages are based on the body weight of the patient. If the patient is a child, body weight is particularly crucial since children's weight varies so much. Don't forget that you would record the weight of a child on a centile chart.

 Connections

See *2.6 Giving medication* (p. 45) for more on drug dosages.

Height
One of the clichés of romantic fiction is the tall, dark, handsome stranger – well, if he were 6 feet 2 inches tall he'd be '1 metre 88' or 1.88 metres (1.88m) in metric.

1.88m means 1 whole metre, 8 tenths of a metre and 8 hundredths of a metre. In practical terms, this means 1 metre 88 centimetres, or 188 centimetres.

Someone 5 feet 3 inches tall is '1 metre 60', or 1.6 metres, or 160 centimetres.

In fact, we tend to judge other people's height in relation to our own. The easiest way to become familiar with heights in metric is to measure yourself in metric and 'think metric' when you're looking at other people. Start by recording your height in metric in your maths diary.

These days, adult patients' heights are not normally measured as a routine; however, children's heights are measured and recorded according to local practice – this may mean that the height is recorded and plotted on the centile chart, or a note might be entered in the child's records together with the date.

 Practice tip

Accurate measurement and recording of weight is important:

- to monitor growth in children
- to calculate drug dosage
- to assess the dosage of anaesthetics
- to monitor the retention and output of bodily fluids.

Activities – Working with height and weight

Task 1

Make a list of some co-operative friends or family members, preferably including children. Estimate their heights in metres and centimetres and their weights in kilograms. Measure them to check your estimates.

Task 2

Tomorrow, note all the references to metres, centimetres and kilograms that you come across in your maths diary.

Task 3

A 1.52m-tall woman with a serious heart condition weighed 70kg on admission to hospital. She was put on a special diet and is losing weight at a rate of 3kg each week. If she continues to lose weight at this rate, how long will it take her to reach a target weight in the acceptable range 38–55kg?

Task 4

A boy, 78cm tall, weighed 7kg on admission to hospital. The acceptable range is 8.8–12.4kg. Was he overweight or underweight?
Note: The boy's height is given in centimetres because he is less than one metre tall. The same height could be written in metres as 0.78m.

Task 5

If a patient's weight is written '13.59kg', how would you say that in kilograms and grams? How much does the patient weigh to the nearest kilogram?

 Connections

See 'Rounding off decimals' in *3.3 Decimals and fractions* (p. 79) if you're not sure.

Task 6

A child weighing 20kg is prescribed cefotaxime (a broad-spectrum antibiotic) daily in four equally divided doses. Dosage is 100mg/kg (100 milligrams of drug per kilogram of the patient's body weight). How much should the child be given in each dose?

▶ 2.3 The fluid balance chart

Recording a patient's details on a fluid balance chart means that you measure and record the fluid intake and output accurately over a 24-hour period using the '24-hour clock'.

 Connections

Unsure? Turn to *3.7 The 24-hour clock* (p. 98).

Intake and output of fluids

There are various routes by which a patient takes in fluid:

- orally
- intravenously (IV)
- subcutaneously
- rectally.

Conversely the patient may lose fluids in the form of:

- urine
- vomit
- wound drainage
- blood loss
- stools (faeces)
- perspiration.

Some of these outputs, such as urine, vomit and wound drainage, can be measured accurately; others, such as perspiration and fluid loss in the stools, cannot be measured accurately and easily and therefore estimates have to be made.

The amount of fluid intake depends on the condition of the patient and whether fluids are restricted or extra fluids are needed. A dehydrated patient, for example, would need to be given extra fluids either by increasing her oral intake or by giving fluids intravenously or subcutaneously. A patient with heart or renal disease might be on restricted fluids. Either way, it is essential that the fluid balance chart is kept accurately to avoid a potentially dangerous misdiagnosis and treatment.

Activities – Working with the fluid balance chart

Use the fluid balance chart to record the information given in the following tasks:

Task 1

Dorothy Green is prescribed 1 litre (1 000ml) of dextrose 5%+KCl (potassium chloride) over 6 hours to start at 0800 hours. After 4 hours, at which point 550ml has been infused, the doctor changes the prescription to 1 litre normal saline over 12 hours. At midnight 950ml has been infused. What is Ms Green's total intravenous fluid intake in the period from 0800 hours to midnight?

Task 2

At 0800 hours Ms Green has a cup of tea (150ml), at 1200 hours she has a glass of orange juice (180ml), at 1500 hours and again at 1900 hours she has a cup of tea. How much fluid has she taken orally altogether?

Task 3

Ms Green's urine output is 200ml at 0900 hours, 300ml at 1600 hours and 150ml at 2000 hours. How much urine has she passed altogether?

Task 4

Work out Ms Green's total fluid intake and output from 0800 hours.

Task 5

How could the design of this fluid balance chart be improved? Design your own chart, noting your reasons for any changes in your maths diary.

▶ 2.4   Nutrition

Nutrition plays an important part in the recovery of the patient.

Nutritional assessment should therefore be seen as an important aspect when planning total patient care since an unbalanced or inadequate diet may lead to complications and delay recovery.

The term 'malnutrition' refers to both under- and over-nutrition. Under-nutrition in older people has been highlighted in recent literature and government policy documents as a major cause for concern (BAPEN, 2004).

The fluid balance chart

MR/MRS/MISS/MS:
SURNAME:
FORENAMES:
PATIENT NUMBER:
CONSULTANT:
WARD:
DATE:

OTHER INSTRUCTIONS

TIME	I.V. INPUT							ORAL/N.G. INPUT		OUTPUT URINE/SECRETIONS/DRAINAGE					
	1			2				Oral	Running Total	Urine		1		2	
	Blood Plasma	Type	Vol	Running Total	Type	Vol	Running Total				Running Total		Running Total		Running Total
01.00															
02.00															
03.00															
04.00															
05.00															
06.00															
07.00															
08.00															
09.00															

10.00												
11.00												
12.00												
13.00												
14.00												
15.00												
16.00												
17.00												
18.00												
19.00												
20.00												
21.00												
22.00												
23.00												
00.00												
TOTALS												

TOTAL INTAKE ml.

TOTAL OUTPUT ml.

TOTAL BALANCE/24 HRS =

MINUS INSENSIBLE LOSS =

Over-nutrition is also becoming a serious health problem for all age groups, especially for children, who may experience long-term damage caused by obesity in childhood.

A multi-professional approach involving the nurse, doctor, dietician, speech therapist and the patient's relative or carer is required when establishing nutritional status in order to provide appropriately for the nutritional requirements of the patient. It is essential that during the assessment stage a dietary history is taken which includes the patient's present dietary preferences, any eating problems or restrictions and potential dietary needs.

Accurate measurement of a patient's weight on admission to hospital is usually required so that, if necessary, a comparison may be made between the patient's usual weight (if known) and actual weight.

Body mass index

Body mass index (BMI) is used to determine whether or not an individual's weight is within the range considered to be healthy. It works on the basis of the relationship between an individual's weight and height.

For patients for whom it is difficult to obtain an accurate measure of height by direct measurement, alternative suggestions for estimating height are made in MUST (the Malnutrition Universal Screening Tool; see p. 41). These include estimating height from the length of the patient's ulna and estimating the patient's BMI category from his or her mid-upper-arm circumference (MUAC). The MUST Explanatory Booklet gives details of other alternative measurements (knee height and demispan) that can also be used to estimate height (BAPEN, 2004).

Here we suggest you use yourself as a guinea pig to work out your body mass index:

1   Measure your height in metres and multiply the figure by itself (i.e. square your height).
2   Weigh yourself in kilograms.
3   Divide your weight by your height squared.

This can be written as a formula:

$$\text{BMI} = \frac{\text{weight (kg)}}{\text{height (m)}^2}$$

For example, if you are 1.6m (5 feet 3 inches) tall and weigh 65kg (10 stone), this is the calculation you would do:

Square your height: $1.6 \times 1.6 = 2.56$
Divide your weight by your height squared: $65 \div 2.56 = 25.39$
The answer is your BMI: 25 (correct to the nearest whole number)

These are the recommended BMI categories for a healthy adult, as set out by the government's Food Standards Agency:[3]

below 20	underweight
20–24.9	ideal
25–29.9	overweight
30–39.9	obese
over 40	extremely obese

The Food Standards Agency website includes an interactive BMI calculator.

BMI is only a guideline and it's only one measure of health. Body fat percentage, blood pressure, resting heart rate, cholesterol and other measurements are also important.

Examples
If a man weighs 70kg and is 1.73m tall, his height squared is 1.73×1.73 square metres (m^2). His BMI is:

$$\text{BMI} = \frac{70}{2.99} = 23.4$$

A woman weighing 50kg whose height is 1.78m:
Height squared is 1.78×1.78 square metres $= 3.17m^2$.

$$\text{BMI} = \frac{50}{3.17} = 15.8$$

A woman weighing 76kg, whose height is 1.65m:
Height squared is 1.65×1.65 square metres $= 2.72m^2$.

$$\text{BMI} = \frac{50}{2.72} = 18.4$$

A man weighing 105kg, whose height is 1.75m:
Height squared is 1.75×1.75 square metres $= 3.1m^2$.

$$\text{BMI} = \frac{105}{3.1} = 33.8$$

---

3 Food Standards Agency (http://www.food.gov.uk/); see also http://www.food.gov.uk/healthiereating/are_you_healthyweight/bmi_calc).

Body Surface Area estimates

Body Surface Area estimates are also used for drug calculation purposes, especially in paediatric medicine. You work out a patient's Body Surface Area by means of a graph called a nomogram (see, for example, Insley, 1996), or the BNF Calculator (http://bnf.org/bnf/extra/current/noframes/450018.htm), which relate the patient's height or length, weight and surface area according to a set formula.

The Malnutrition Universal Screening Tool (MUST)

The Malnutrition Universal Screening Tool (MUST) is a five-step screening tool to identify adults who are malnourished, at risk of malnutrition (undernutrition) or obese. In addition to the patient's BMI score, weight loss and the effect of any acute disease are taken into account in MUST. It includes management guidelines which can be used to develop a care plan. It is designed for use in hospitals, community and other care settings by all care workers. MUST enables the healthcare professional to make an informed risk assessment for the patient. Reassessment will be required as the patient's circumstances change.[4]

In summary, the five MUST steps are:

- Step 1   Measure height and weight to get a BMI score using chart provided. If unable to obtain height and weight, use the alternative procedures shown in the MUST guide.
- Step 2   Note percentage unplanned weight loss and score using tables provided.
- Step 3   Establish acute disease effect and score.
- Step 4   Add scores from steps 1, 2 and 3 together to obtain overall risk of malnutrition.
- Step 5   Use management guidelines and/or local policy to develop care plan.

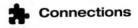 **Connections**

See *2.2 Measuring weight and height* (p. 27) for more on this.

---

4 The full MUST guide is available to download as a pdf file from BAPEN (www.bapen.org.uk).

'Malnutrition Universal Screening Tool' ('MUST') M A G

BAPEN
dvancing Clinical Nutrition

Malnutrition Advisory Group
A Standing Committee of BAPEN

BAPEN is registered charity number 1023927   www.bapen.org.uk

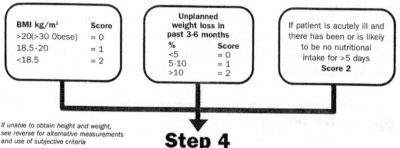

Step 1   +   Step 2   +   Step 3
BMI score   Weight loss score   Acute disease effect score

BMI kg/m²	Score
>20(>30 Obese)	= 0
18.5-20	= 1
<18.5	= 2

Unplanned weight loss in past 3-6 months

%	Score
<5	= 0
5-10	= 1
>10	= 2

If patient is acutely ill and there has been or is likely to be no nutritional intake for >5 days
Score 2

If unable to obtain height and weight, see reverse for alternative measurements and use of subjective criteria

Step 4
Overall risk of malnutrition

Add Scores together to calculate overall risk of malnutrition
Score 0 Low Risk   Score 1 Medium Risk   Score 2 or more High Risk

Step 5
Management guidelines

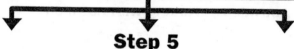

0
Low Risk
Routine clinical care

- Repeat screening
  Hospital – weekly
  Care Homes – monthly
  Community – annually
  for special groups
  e.g. those >75 yrs

1
Medium Risk
Observe

- Document dietary intake for 3 days if subject in hospital or care home

- If improved or adequate intake – little clinical concern; if no improvement – clinical concern - follow local policy

- Repeat screening
  Hospital – weekly
  Care Home – at least monthly
  Community – at least every 2-3 months

2 or more
High Risk
Treat*

- Refer to dietitian, Nutritional Support Team or implement local policy
- Improve and increase overall nutritional intake
- Monitor and review care plan
  Hospital – weekly
  Care Home – monthly
  Community – monthly

* Unless detrimental or no benefit is expected from nutritional support e.g. imminent death.

All risk categories:
- Treat underlying condition and provide help and advice on food choices, eating and drinking when necessary.
- Record malnutrition risk category.
- Record need for special diets and follow local policy.

Obesity:
- Record presence of obesity. For those with underlying conditions, these are generally controlled before the treatment of obesity.

Re-assess subjects identified at risk as they move through care settings
See The 'MUST' Explanatory Booklet for further details and The 'MUST' Report for supporting evidence.

Food and energy

Food is required, among other things, for energy. Energy requirements vary according to the patient's age, sex and level of physical activity.

You have probably heard of calories (also known as small calories) as a measure of the energy value of food. You may also have heard of kilocalories (kcal), also known as kilogram calories or Calories (Cal), which are 1 000 times larger than small calories. Both calories and kilocalories have largely been replaced by the metric (SI) unit used to measure potential energy in food, the joule (J). You will normally come across the joule in the form of the kilojoule (kJ). A kilojoule is 1 000 times larger than a joule.

A large banana has 80 kilocalories or 334 kilojoules.

 Connections

See *3.8 Conversions* (p. 99) for information on converting from kilocalories to kilojoules and vice versa.

 Activities – Working with nutrition

Task 1

For every packet or tin of food you buy in the next week, write down the nutritional information printed on the labels in your maths diary and

(a) take note of how foods differ in their energy values

(b) identify one high- and one low-energy food and record their energy values.

Task 2

Choose one of your patients who is on a special diet. Talk to a dietician about the patient's 24-hour food energy intake. Record this information in your maths diary.

Task 3

Estimate the food energy present in the following meals (assume standard helpings):

(a) two small slices of wholemeal bread with butter and jam and a cup of tea without sugar

(b) rice with grilled chicken and lettuce.

Task 4

Now try these:

1 A patient weighs 65kg and is 1.73m tall. What is her BMI?
2 A patient weighs 92kg and is 1.83m tall. What is his BMI?
3 A patient weighs 110kg and is 1.68m tall. What is her BMI?
4 A patient weighs 50kg and is 1.72m tall. What is his BMI?
5 A patient weighs 55kg and is 1.62m tall. He has pneumonia. Use MUST to identify the patient's level of risk.
6 A patient weighs 84kg and is 1.90m tall. He has lost 7kg in the last 5 months. Use MUST to identify his level of risk.
7 A patient weighs 73kg and is 1.58m tall. She has a urinary tract infection and has lost 11kg in the last 6 months. Use MUST to identify her level of risk.

▶ 2.5   Infant feeding

Prepacked foods are now available in most paediatric units in hospitals, but as a nurse you will need to have some knowledge of the calculation of infant feeds in relation to body weight.

Calculating a baby's expected weight

As a starting point when calculating a baby's expected weight, you need to know the birth weight and the baby's age in weeks. Also you need to remember that a baby may lose and then regain up to one-tenth ($\frac{1}{10}$) or 10% of body weight during the first two weeks of life, for example, a baby weighing 3000 grams at birth may lose up to 300 grams. Some babies may lose less, while others may not lose any weight at all. Babies who lose more than 10% of their birth weight should be carefully monitored.

 Connections

Look again at the centile chart. Centile charts are a useful guide to weight gain and loss in children.
If you need help with percentages, turn to *3.4 Percentages* (p. 88).
For grams and kilograms, turn to *3.6 The metric (SI) system* (p. 94).

Babies generally regain their birth weight by the end of the second week, double their birth weight at around 5 months old and treble it at around one year old. Average weight gain is approximately 200 grams per week during the first year of life. Therefore a 10-week-old baby who weighed 3 000 grams (3 kilograms) at birth would have an expected weight of 4 600 grams or 4.6 kilograms.

This is calculated as follows:

The baby is 10 weeks old – but remember that babies first lose weight and then regain their birth weight in the first two weeks, so at 10 weeks old the baby should have gained 8 times 200 grams ($8 \times 200g = 1\,600g$).

Add the expected weight gain (1 600 grams) to the baby's birth weight to get the expected weight of the baby at 10 weeks ($3\,000 + 1600 = 4\,600g$).

4 600 grams is the same as 4.6 kilograms because 1 000 grams make 1 kilogram.

Fluid and energy requirement

In addition to the baby's expected weight, you will need to know how much fluid and energy intake the baby requires daily.

Normal healthy babies generally need approximately 200 millilitres per kilogram (200ml/kg) of body weight per day. Therefore for a baby weighing 3 kilograms, the fluid intake per day should be:

$3 \times 200ml = 600ml$ of fluid per day.

The energy intake is approximately 540 kilojoules per kilogram (540kJ/kg) of body weight per day. The same baby, weighing 3kg, will therefore need an energy intake of:

$3 \times 540kJ = 1\,620kJ$ per day.

The total amount for the day is divided into equal amounts for each feed. The number of feeds will vary from baby to baby; some babies are fed at four-hourly intervals (six times a day) for the first few months; others are fed on demand.

Activities – Working with infant feeding

Task 1

A baby weighed 3kg at birth. By the beginning of week two the baby's weight had dropped to 2.8kg.

(a)   Is this within the acceptable range?

(b)   How much weight has the baby lost?

(c)   What would the normal weight loss be for a baby of this birth weight?

Task 2

What is the expected weight of an 8-week-old baby who weighed 3.5kg at birth?

Task 3

A baby boy weighs 2.5kg at birth. At the end of the first week he weighs 1.9kg. Would this give you cause for concern?

Task 4

What is the total fluid and energy required per day for a 10-week-old baby weighing 5kg?

Task 5

How much fluid and energy should a baby weighing 6kg be given in each feed if she is fed six times a day?

Task 6

How much fluid and energy should a baby weighing 3kg be given in each feed if he is fed at four-hourly intervals?

▶ 2.6   Giving medication

Medication is administered in various ways which are divided into two categories: parenterally (meaning administered in any way other than by mouth) and non-parenterally or orally (meaning administered by mouth).

When you give medication orally in tablet or liquid form, you can easily check whether you're in the right range:

- tablets are generally taken as 1 to 2 tablets
- liquid doses are generally in the range 1ml to 20ml.

You need to take note of the unit in which the drug is supplied (100mg tablet, 200mg capsule, etc.) and the strength of the drug in its different forms.

The formula is:

$$\text{what you want} = \frac{\text{what you need}}{\text{what you've got}}$$

This can also be expressed as:

$$\text{amount required} = \frac{\text{amount prescribed}}{\substack{\text{amount in each tablet, capsule or} \\ \text{standard liquid measure}}}$$

Tablets may be halved or quartered (*if they have a score mark; not if they don't*), but they should not be crushed, nor should capsules be opened, as this renders the drug off-licence and you would be liable for any damage to the patient. If the patient refuses to take tablets, check with the pharmacist to see if the drug is available in liquid or other forms.

Drugs are normally packaged with adults in mind. In the case of some specified drugs for adults and children, recommended drug dosage is calculated according to BMI or Body Surface Area estimates.

In some drugs, the dosage varies according to age and/or body mass. For example, the dose of Penicillin V for children is age-related: for a child up to one year old it is 62.5mg qds; for ages 1 to 5 years it is 125mg qds; and for ages 6 to 12,250mg qds.

Older people are more likely to be prescribed several drugs to treat different diseases. This increases the risk of adverse drug actions and interactions, including the risk of falls. Some older people find it difficult to swallow tablets and if tablets are prescribed, it is important that sufficient water is taken to avoid ulceration in the digestive tract. Alternative forms of medication, such as liquid, should be considered in these cases.

For more information, see the *British National Formulary* (*BNF*). See also the Introduction to this book for information on how experienced nurses calculate error-critical drug dosages.

Decimals in medication
You will come across quantities of drugs recorded as numbers including decimals, such as Digoxin 62.5 micrograms. But what does the 62.5 mean?

Start with what you know: whole numbers.

Any numbers to the left of the decimal point are whole numbers, in this case sixty-two (62) micrograms.

Any numbers to the right of the decimal point mean less than one microgram. Here there is a 5 to the right of the decimal point (.5).

A number immediately next to the decimal point on the right indicates the number of tenths. In other words, .5 means five-tenths $(\frac{5}{10})$, which is the same as one half $(\frac{1}{2})$ of a microgram.

Digoxin 62.5 micrograms means sixty-two and a half micrograms of digoxin is contained in each tablet.

Similarly, glibenclamide 2.5mg means that two and a half milligrams of the drug is contained in each tablet.

 ## Connections

If you're unsure about decimals, work through the section on decimals in *3.3 Decimals and fractions* (p. 79).

Look at this example:

> 5ml of Simple Linctus BP consists of:
> citric acid monohydrate 125mg
> concentrated anise water 0.05ml
> chloroform spirit 0.3ml
> amaranth solution 0.075ml
> syrup to 5ml

'Syrup to 5ml' means that the sample of solution is made up to 5ml by adding syrup.

As you see, a preparation such as Simple Linctus BP does not only consist of the active ingredients – for example, this linctus has a high sugar content and would not be suitable for someone with diabetes.

Look at the decimals. The linctus contains 0.3ml of chloroform spirit, 0.05ml of concentrated anise water, and 0.075ml of amaranth solution. The 0.3ml of chloroform spirit indicates that there are three-tenths of a millilitre of chloroform spirit in the 5ml sample of linctus. The 0.05 means that there are five-hundredths of a millilitre of concentrated anise water because the second figure to the right of the decimal point means hundredths. Similarly, there are seventy-five-thousandths of a millilitre of amaranth solution.

Note that these ingredients, and the syrup, are listed by volume, in milli-litres. By contrast, the citric acid monohydrate is listed by weight (125mg); it is dissolved in the liquid which is made up to 5ml so the 125mg is *included* in the total volume (5ml), not added to it (see *3.5 Ratios* (p. 92) for more on this).

Non-medical prescribing

Non-medical prescribing may be done by both supplementary prescribers and independent nurse prescribers. Supplementary prescribers include pharmacists and nurses in partnership with an independent prescriber, i.e. a doctor or dentist,[5] with the agreement of the patient. Independent nurse prescribers take responsibility for clinical assessment, diagnosis and clinical management of the patient, prescribing where necessary. The range of products that an independent nurse prescriber may prescribe is limited under law. There are two formularies from which nurses can prescribe, depending on their qualification. Health visitors and district nurses can prescribe from the *Nurse Prescribers' Formulary* which can be found in the appendixes and indexes section of the *BNF*. Nurses who have competed the Extended Nurse Prescribing course can prescribe from a greater range of medicines but only for specific indications (see the *British National Formulary* for a full list).

Non-medical prescribers need to be aware of the range of strengths of medication available and the different forms and routes, e.g. liquid, tablets, injections, etc. They need to consider what is the appropriate strength and form to give, for example, 2×2.5mg or 1×5mg. Consideration may have to be given as to the size of the tablet and the ease of swallowing for some patients. It is worth noting that it is usually more cost-effective to prescribe a higher dose, i.e. 1×5mg rather than 2×2.5mg.

Prescribers also need to be aware of differences in bioavailability (i.e. how much drug is available in the body to act) between different forms; for example, digoxin 62.5 micrograms in tablet form is equivalent to 50 micrograms in liquid form. Also, Lithium carbonate 200mg tablet is equiv-alent to Lithium citrate 509 milligrams in liquid form.

Non-medical prescribers also need to consider the difference between various modified-release preparations and the effect of these on frequency of dosage. For example, MST (Morphine sulphate tablets) should be prescribed as a twice-daily dose as opposed to MXL (Morphine

---

5 Podiatrists, physiotherapists, optometrists and radiographers will shortly be included as supplementary prescribers.

sulphate capsule), which should be prescribed once daily. Similarly, Adalat LA is prescribed once daily, while Adalat Retard is prescribed twice daily.

Remember that your local pharmacist will be able to give you advice and guidance on all the above issues on form, strength and dosage.

Drug packaging

There is no standard 'month' in drug packaging: some manufacturers package drugs for 28 days; others for 30 days. For example, Paroxetine and Fluoxetine are available in packs of 30, as opposed to Citalopram and Sertraline, which are available in packs of 28. This may cause difficulties when prescribing equivalent quantities of different medicines. 28 days' supply is generally accepted as best practice; however, 56 days' supply is often chosen for repeat prescriptions for the convenience of the patient and the prescriber.

To ensure drugs are prescribed in equivalent quantities, put down full directions, including the number of days' supply, in the box on the FP10 (prescription form) or against each item, in which case the pharmacist will do the calculations.

For example, 1/52 indicates one week's supply; 28/7 indicates 28 days' supply; and 1/12 indicates one month's supply (the pharmacist will then decide whether to supply 28 or 30 days' worth of medication).

Alternatively, prescriptions may be written as follows:

For once a day ($\dot{\text{I}}$ od) medication, prescribe 28 tablets.

For 1 tablet twice a day ($\dot{\text{I}}$ bd) prescribe 56 tablets.

For 2 tablets once a day ($\ddot{\text{I}}\ddot{\text{I}}$ od) prescribe 56 tablets.

For 1 tablet three times a day ($\dot{\text{I}}$ tds) prescribe 84 tablets.

For 1 tablet four times a day ($\dot{\text{I}}$ qds) prescribe 112 tablets.

For 2 tablets three times a day ($\ddot{\text{I}}\ddot{\text{I}}$ tds) prescribe 168 tablets.

For 2 tablets four times a day ($\ddot{\text{I}}\ddot{\text{I}}$ qds) prescribe 224 tablets.

Inhalers

It is important to be aware of the dose unit for inhalers in order to be able to prescribe the correct quantity. For example, Salbutamol comes in 200-

dose units so if the patient is having 8 units per day (2 puffs, 4 times a day) which would be 8 units per day, that means the patient would need 224 units for 28 days. The prescription would need to be for more than one inhaler as one inhaler only contains 200 dose units.

Dermatological preparations
Dermatological preparations must be prescribed in sufficient quantity to ensure their effectiveness. Suitable quantities are listed in the *BNF* under 'Management of Skin Conditions'. These recommendations do not apply to cortico-steroid preparations.

Intravenous (IV) drug administration
There are different methods by which drugs may be administered intra-venously. Which method you use depends on the volume of fluid to be infused, the type of drug and the condition of the patient.

Drugs may be administered intravenously by:

(a) *continuous* infusion – when a large volume of fluid is required over a 24-hour period
(b) *intermittent* transfusion – *either* when a smaller volume is infused over a short period and requested at intervals during the 24-hour period *or* direct intermittent administration, when the drug is given directly into a vein using a needle and syringe or via a canula. This method is used when a maximum concentration of the drug is required quickly.

Calculating the rate of IV administration
IV is calculated in rates per minute. There are different types of infusion sets which deliver at 10, 15, 20 and 60 drops per millilitre (drops/ml).

These are the things you should consider when calculating infusion rates:

- which infusion set is being used
- the amount to be infused
- the time period over which the drug is to be infused.

This is the formula for calculating infusion rates (i.e. working out how many drops you need per minute): multiply the drops per millilitre by the amount to be infused and divide by the total time. You can write this like this (remember that the horizontal line means 'divide the top numbers by the bottom numbers'):

$$\frac{\text{drops per millilitre of the giving set x amount to be infused in ml}}{\text{total time of infusion in minutes}}$$

Therefore, if a patient has to have 1000ml of 5% dextrose over 10 hours using a 15 drops per millilitre infusion set, you calculate:

$$\frac{15 \text{ drops per millilitre of the giving set} \times 1000\text{ml to be infused}}{10 \text{ hours x } 60 \text{ minutes}}$$

$$= \frac{15 \times 1\,000}{600} = 25 \text{ drops per minute}$$

Activities – Working with medication

Task 1
The doctor prescribed 10ml of magnesium trisilicate three times a day. How many standard 5ml spoonsful do you need for each dose?

Task 2
Aspirin is dispensed in 300mg tablets. How many tablets would you need for a dose of 900mg?

Probably the quickest way to deal with this is to try a few likely answers. Three hundred . . . nine hundred? Looks like 3 tablets?
3 tablets with 300mg in each would give you 900mg, so that's right.

Task 3
You need to give 1.5g of robaxin and 500mg tablets are available. How many tablets do you need?

You can't easily compare 1.5g with 500mg because the units are different. Rewrite 1.5g as 1 500mg, and think again. Try a few likely answers: you need 1 500mg and each tablet has 500mg. Fifteen hundred . . . five hundred? Four tablets? Four tablets with 500mg in each would be 4 x 500, i.e. 2 000mg. Too big, probably 3? Three tablets with 500mg in each would give you 3 x 500 =1 500mg, so that's right.

Look back at the ingredients of Simple Linctus BP (p. 47) for the next three tasks:

Task 4   Recognition
Which ingredients of Simple Linctus BP are listed by volume, and which are listed by weight?

Task 5   Calculation

The normal adult dose of Simple Linctus BP is 5ml, 3–4 times daily; how much would a patient on this dose take in a day?

Task 6   Metric measurement

(a) What is the main constituent of the linctus by volume?
(b) List the following in order by volume, largest first: concentrated anise water 0.05ml; chloroform spirit 0.3ml; amaranth solution 0.075ml.

Task 7

An anti-inflammatory analgesic, ibuprofen, is prescribed for a woman in a dose of 1.8g daily in three divided doses, after food. Each tablet contains 200mg. How many tablets should be given at each dose?

Task 8

Risperidone is dispensed in 1mg tablets. How many tablets are needed for a dose of 6mg per day in two divided doses?

Task 9

A slow intravenous injection of 250–500mg aminophylline 25mg/ml is prescribed. How much would you give to a patient weighing 55kg if the dose is 5mg/kg?

Task 10

Bisacodyl is available in suppositories containing 5mg. How many should you give if 10mg is prescribed?

Task 11

Hydrocortisone (as sodium succinate) comes in a 100mg vial (with a 2ml ampoule of water) for reconstitution for administration by injection. How many vials would be required for a dose of 200mg three times in 24 hours?

Task 12

A drug is given in 2% solution. What does this mean?

Task 13

A patient has to have 500ml of normal saline over 5 hours using 10 drops per millilitre infusion set. Calculate the infusion rate.

Task 14

A patient has to have 1000ml of dextrose over 8 hours using 60 drops per millilitre infusion set. Calculate the infusion rate.

If you end up with a whole number and a fraction, just round your answer to the nearest whole number. For example, $3\frac{1}{10}$ is only just over 3 while $3\frac{7}{10}$ is nearly 4.

 ## Connections

If you need more help with fractions, turn to *3.3 Decimals and fractions* (p. 79).

▶ 2.7   Staffing and budget calculations

A budget is a statement of planned income and expenditure over an agreed period, usually a year (the 'financial year').

The responsibility for managing budgets within the National Health Service is now devolved to individual service managers, something which is common practice in the private sector. As a healthcare professional in the public or private sector, therefore, you will be expected to work within a delegated budget and you might also be involved in developing strategic plans for your work area. You will need to be able to handle the calculations involved in budgeting with confidence in order to ensure that you get the best value from the resources available. This section is intended to introduce you to some of the basics of budget calculations; for greater depth and detail, see one of the books available, such as *Budgeting Skills: A Guide For Nurse Managers* (Taylor, 1992) or *The NHS Budget-Holder's Survival Guide* (Bailey, 1994).

You need to understand how the budget is set out and to be able to do the necessary calculations. Here are some points you would need to consider if you were analysing your budget:

- What is the total annual budget for the financial year in terms of revenue (income) and expenditure (costs, both pay and non-pay)?
- *Staffing calculations are an important aspect of budgeting since the pay element is usually the largest part of the healthcare budget. Staffing levels are measured in Whole Time Equivalents (WTEs).*

 ## Connections

For more on staffing, see *3.5 Ratios* (p. 92).

- What is included in the budget? For example, are capital costs included? Capital costs would include such things as the cost of the purchase of additional land or buildings. You need to remember that additional capital expenditure may have implications for running costs in the short or long term.
- Is your unit expected to break even, make a profit or to remain within budget?
- When does the financial year begin and end?
  The financial year usually runs from April to March.
- What is the range of services you will be expected to provide? Are any of your services expected to produce added value?
- Is there a predetermined dependency level?
- *The number of healthcare staff required for a given number of patients in a given situation is known as the 'dependency level'.*
- Is there a contingency fund to cover emergencies such as staff sickness?
- Is there an investment programme and, if so, what is it and over what period does it operate?
- What, if any, facilities are bought in and what resources are allocated to cover these?

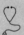 **Practice tip**

Remember that the mathematics of budgeting may be quite straightforward – often it involves no more than simple arithmetic. Identify the assistance that is available to you as a manager in the form of administrative and professional support and information technology and develop a system whereby you are able to keep track of income and expenditure.

 Activities – Working with budgets

Task 1

You are the manager of a 50-bed nursing home which has 40 single rooms and 10 twin rooms. If the home is running at full occupancy, how much weekly income is generated if the income for each single-bedded room is £325 per week and that for each occupant of a twin-bedded room is £300 per week?

○ ○ ▷

Task 2

The dependency levels in your unit increase: what is the increase in costs if you have to employ an additional Registered nurse at a cost of £7 per hour for each of three 8-hour shifts daily for one week?

Task 3

If the non-pay budget of a private clinic is £200 000, the pay budget is £500 000 and you do not use your contingency budget:

(a) how much profit would you make if the estimated annual income is £1 000 000?
(b) what is your profit, expressed as a percentage of the income received?

 Connections

Unsure of percentages? Turn to *3.4 Percentages* (p. 88).

Task 4

Calculate the hours and Whole Time Equivalents of a clerical officer in the following examples, assuming 1 clerical WTE = 35 hours per week.

17.5 hours = _____ WTE   0.75 WTE = _____ hours

14 hours = _____ WTE   0.25 WTE = _____ hours

 Connections

If you need to refresh your memory on decimals, turn to *3.3 Decimals and fractions* (p. 79).

Task 5

Calculate the following nursing hours and WTEs, assuming one nursing WTE is 37.5 hours:

0.5 WTE   = _____ hours per week

0.75 WTE   = _____ hours per week

12 hours per week = _____ WTE

9 hours per week = _____ WTE

Annual leave calculations

In calculating annual leave you need to be systematic.

First establish what the annual leave entitlement is for full-time workers in the area of healthcare with which you are concerned. Working hours and leave entitlements vary, for example, for nurses in the NHS: 'full time' normally means 37.5 hours per week and the holiday entitlement is around 28 days. For most other staff, full-time working varies from 36 to 40 hours. Junior doctors work the longest hours; however, a European directive now requires that they do not work more than 48 hours per week.

To work out the number of days' annual leave entitlement, multiply the number of hours worked by the full-time annual leave entitlement and then divide by the number of full-time hours. If the answer comes to, say, 13.75 days, round off (in this case to 14 days). However, if the answer comes to 13.5 days, leave it as it is, since annual leave may be taken in half days.

For example, if a cleaner works part time for 18 hours a week and the full-time annual leave entitlement is 28 days for a 37.5-hour working week, then you can set out the calculation like this:

$$\text{Annual leave entitlement} = \frac{18 \text{ hours} \times 28 \text{ days}}{37.5 \text{ hours}} = \frac{504}{37.5}$$
$$= 13.44 \text{ days}$$
$$= 13.5 \text{ days}$$

13.44 days is rounded up to 13.5 for practical purposes.

For a nurse working part time for 30 hours a week, annual leave entitlement may be calculated as follows:

$$\text{Annual leave entitlement} = \frac{30 \text{ hours} \times 28 \text{ days}}{37.5 \text{ hours}} = \frac{840}{37.5}$$
$$= 22.4 \text{ days}$$
$$= 22.5 \text{ days}$$

Again, 22.4 days is rounded up to 22.5 for practical purposes.

A junior doctor's full-time hours are 48 hours per week and annual leave entitlement is 30 days, so a junior doctor working part time, 40 hours a week, will be entitled to:

$$\frac{40 \text{ hours} \times 30 \text{ days (full-time entitlement)}}{48 \text{ hours (full-time hours)}} = \frac{1\,200}{48} = 25 \text{ days' annual leave}$$

A junior doctor working part time, 30 hours a week, will be entitled to:

$$\frac{30 \text{ hours} \times 30 \text{ days}}{48} = \frac{900}{48} = 18.75 = 19 \text{ days (rounded off)}$$

A healthcare assistant working 20 hours per week has a full-time annual leave entitlement of 25 days. Full-time HCA hours are 37.5 per week.

$$\frac{20 \text{ hours} \times 25}{37.5} = \frac{500}{37.5} = 13.3 = 13 \text{ days (rounded off)}$$

For a healthcare assistant working 20 hours per week, the calculation would be:

$$\frac{18 \text{ hours} \times 25}{37.5} = \frac{450}{37.5} = 12 \text{ days}$$

An administrator works 21 hours per week. Full-time hours are 36 hours per week and full-time annual leave entitlement is 27 days:

$$\frac{21 \times 27}{36} = \frac{567}{36} = 15.75 = 16 \text{ days (rounded off)}$$

 Activity

Task 6

Now work out the annual leave entitlement for these workers:

	Part-time hours	Full-time annual leave entitlement	Full-time hours	Annual leave entitlement
1	28	27	36	_____
2	36	30	48	_____
3	18	28	37.5	_____
4	15	28	37.5	_____
5	30	27	36	_____

► 2.8   Demographic profiles

Demographic profiling has become a very important tool in community nursing and the production of a neighbourhood study is now a mandatory part of health visitor training.

The main aim of demographic profiling is the collection of data in order to assess community needs and enable healthcare staff to plan and develop services to meet these needs.

Profiling encourages healthcare professionals to develop a more proactive, collaborative role in health promotion and disease prevention. Priorities may be set, either to meet the needs of the community directly or to highlight deficiencies in service provision and draw managers' attention to them. Profiling may also enable clients to make informed decisions about their own health and wellbeing. Cernik and Wearne (1992: 345) argue that profiling offers health visitors the opportunity to develop progressive primary health care, but point out that, 'like any other tool, a profile is only as effective as the people who use it'. So what makes an effective profile?

What kind of data should I collect?

Communities and their needs vary and so does the data that is collected; there is no set pattern. You need to think about the following questions:

- *Purposes* – what purposes will the profile be put to?
- *Sources* – what sources of information are available? Sources might include, for example, Census returns, voluntary organisations, local authorities, health authorities, public health commissions, surveys, interviews, etc. A useful source of neighbourhood statistics is the Office for National Statistics (ONS) website (http://neighbourhood. statistics.gov.uk/).
- *Analysis* – how are you going to analyse the data after you've collected it? This analysis should produce a clear picture of the health needs of the local community.
- *Comparison* – how does the local community compare with the national picture?

Activities – Working with demographic profiles

Task 1

You are a community health worker (district nurse or health visitor) working in a Well Persons' Clinic. The incidence of high blood pressure in patients coming to the clinic seems to have sharply increased in the last year.

- How would you set about checking whether this is the case?
- How would you record your data?
- What action would you take in relation to other healthcare professionals?
- What advice would you be likely to give to patients?
- What are the implications of sustained high blood pressure for prioritising resources in the clinic?

Task 2

You are undertaking a survey of the provision of residential accommodation for older people and discover that only one black person in a borough with a large number of black residents is living in such residential accommodation. The inference is that black elders are not accessing the provision. Prepare a case to discuss with your manager.

Task 3

The tables below summarise extracts from the 2001 Census Returns for the London Borough of Lewisham. As a health visitor or school or district nurse you need to be able to interpret such tables in order to develop a demographic profile of your area or caseload as a basis for research.

Use the information on the tables below to work out what percentage of the population of the borough is elderly and state how you are defining 'older people'.

Task 4

(a) From the information given in the tables below, can you say how many pensioners in Lewisham live alone?

(b) What percentage is this of the total number of pensioners in Lewisham?

Task 5

Identify a health issue in your specialist area from the Lewisham data and present a case for resources to present to your manager. You might ask for more resources or for the redirection of existing resources.

Area statistics

The following statistics about Lewisham, a borough in south-east London, are based on information from the 2001 Census in England and Wales and, where indicated, the Department for Work and Pensions, the Land Registry and the Home Office.[6]

Resident population and age

The resident population of Lewisham, as measured in the 2001 Census, was 248 922, of which 48% were male and 52% were female.

	Resident population (%)
Under 16	21.1
16–19	4.6
20–29	17.1
30–59	42.7
60–74	9.2
75 and over	5.3
Average age	34.7

Source: 2001 Census, ONS, © Crown Copyright.

Marital status

	Resident population aged 16 and over (%)
Single (never married)	46.0
Married or remarried	35.9
Separated	3.7
Divorced	8.2
Widowed	6.2

Source: 2001 Census, ONS, © Crown Copyright.

---

6 Crown copyright material is reproduced with the permission of the Controller of HMSO and the Queen's Printer for Scotland from: http://neighbourhood.statistics.gov.uk/AreaProfile Frames.asp?PF=Y&AREA=Lewisham&PC=&TID=13&AID=17550.

Ethnic group

Percentage of resident population in ethnic groups	Resident population (%)
White	65.9
of which White Irish	2.8
Mixed	4.2
Asian or Asian British	3.8
Indian	1.4
Pakistani	0.4
Bangladeshi	0.5
Other Asian	1.5
Black or Black British	23.4
Caribbean	12.3
African	9.1
Other Black	2.1
Chinese or Other Ethnic Group	2.7

Source: 2001 Census, ONS, © Crown Copyright.

Religion

	Resident population (%)
Christian	61.2
Buddhist	1.1
Hindu	1.7
Jewish	0.3
Muslim	4.6
Sikh	0.2
Other religions	0.5
No religion	20.4
Religion not stated	10.0

Source: 2001 Census, ONS, © Crown Copyright.

Health and provision of care

The 2001 Census asked people to describe their health over the preceding 12 months as 'good', 'fairly good' or 'not good'.

	Resident population (%)
Good	69.2
Fairly good	22.4
Not good	8.5

Source: 2001 Census, ONS, © Crown Copyright.

Limiting long-term illness, health problem or disability

	Resident population (%)
Had a long-term illness	15.6

Source: 2001 Census, ONS, © Crown Copyright.

Providers of voluntary care

	Resident population (%)
Provided unpaid care	7.9

Source: 2001 Census, ONS, © Crown Copyright.

In August 2000, 7 740 people in Lewisham received the Disability Living Allowance (a benefit paid to people under 65 who are disabled and need help with personal care and/or getting around) (*Source*: Department for Work and Pensions, 2000).

In May 2000, 3 515 people in Lewisham received the Attendance Allowance (paid to people over 65, who are so severely disabled, physically or mentally, that they need supervision or a great deal of help with personal care) (*Source*: Department for Work and Pensions, 2000).

Economic activity

	Resident population aged 16–74 (%)
Employed	59.9
Unemployed	5.6
Economically active full-time students	3.4
Retired	8.7
Economically inactive students	6.5
Looking after home/family	6.5
Permanently sick or disabled	4.8
Economically inactive	4.5

Source: 2001 Census, ONS, © Crown Copyright.

Within Lewisham, 14% of those unemployed were aged 50 and over, 13% had never worked and 34% were long-term unemployed.

In August 2000, there were 7 085 Jobseeker Allowance (JSA) claimants in Lewisham, of which 25% had child dependants. JSA is payable to people under pensionable age who are available for, and actively seeking, work of at least 40 hours a week. These figures refer only to people claiming income-based JSA (*Source*: Department for Work and Pensions, 2000).

In August 2000, there were 22 655 Income Support claimants in Lewisham, of which 2% were aged under 20. Income support can be paid to a person who is aged 16 and over, is not working 16 hours or more a week, and has less money coming in than the law says they need to live on (*Source*: Department for Work and Pensions, 2000).

Students

	Students and schoolchildren aged 16–74
Total number of full-time students and schoolchildren aged 16–74	17 170
Percentage of total resident population	6.9
Total number aged 16–17	4 668
Total number aged 18–74	12 502

Note: Students and schoolchildren were counted at their term-time address.
Source: 2001 Census, ONS, © Crown Copyright.

Qualifications

	Resident population aged 16–74 (%)
Had no qualifications	24.2
Qualified to degree level or higher	29.4

Source: 2001 Census, ONS, © Crown Copyright.

Housing and households
In Lewisham there were 107 412 households in 2001. 99% of the resident population lived in households; the remainder lived in communal establishments.

	Number of households (%)
One-person households	34.8
Pensioners living alone	11.4
Other all-pensioner households	4.6
Contained dependent children	30.4
Lone-parent households with dependent children	10.5
Owner-occupied	50.1
Rented from Council	26.6
Rented from Housing Association or Registered Social Landlord	9.0
Private rented or lived rent free	14.3
Without central heating	9.7
Without sole use of bath, shower or toilet	0.8
Have no car or van	42.8
Have 2 or more cars or vans	13.8
Average household size (number)	2.3
Average number of rooms per household	4.5

Source: 2001 Census, ONS, © Crown Copyright.

Percentage of households living in various types of property

	Number of households (%)
Detached	2.9
Semi-detached	12.9
Terraced	31.5
Flat	52.7

Source: 2001 Census, ONS; The Land Registry, 2001, © Crown Copyright.

Levels of crime in Lewisham

Notifiable offences recorded by the police, April 2000–March 2001

	Violence against the person	Sexual offences	Robbery	Burglary from a dwelling	Theft of a motor vehicle	Theft from a motor vehicle
Total number of offences recorded, Lewisham	5 331	372	1 547	2 494	2 196	2 240
Rate per 1 000 population, Lewisham	21.7	1.5	6.3	10.2	8.9	9.1
Rate per 1 000 population, England and Wales	11.4	0.7	1.8	7.6	6.4	11.9

Source: Home Office, © Crown Copyright.

Part three
Maths refreshers

▶ **Introduction**

This part of the book is designed to refresh your memory of maths, to fill any gaps in your knowledge and understanding and to build on your experience using informal methods that you can do in your head as well as using pen and paper or a calculator.

The maths covered ranges from a fresh look at whole numbers, through the 'four rules' of arithmetic (addition, subtraction, multiplication and division); decimals and fractions; percentages; ratios; the metric system; the 24-hour clock and conversions between metric and imperial measurements of height and weight, between degrees Celsius and degrees Fahrenheit and between calories and kilojoules.

Before you start, look back at *Part one: Learning and you*. There we advised you to:

- share strategies for working out maths problems – remember there's nearly always more than one way of doing a mathematical operation and the 'right' way is the way that works. It's also a good idea to double-check your answer using a different method;
- talk through your feelings about maths – if something doesn't feel right to you, even if you know it gives the correct answer, talk it over with your learning partner and you may find that a different way of looking at the problem helps you to see it more clearly;
- talk over the situations you come across that involve maths, especially those which involve doing maths under pressure, and share strategies for remaining calm and doing the maths.

Use your maths diary to record your feelings about the maths you do and to note down points to remember. Compare notes with your learning partner. Above all, relax and take your time. The more you think about what you're doing and why, and the more you practise, the more thoroughly you will understand and the more confident you will be in the maths in your life.

▶ **3.1   Whole numbers**

Whole numbers (also known as integers) are so familiar that you may feel it's unnecessary to dwell on them. However, it's a good idea to start with what you know and see what you can learn from it.

For example, look closely at 426. You know it means four hundred and twenty-six, but have you ever wondered why?

The reason is that numbers are organised according to a principle called *place value*. Place value means that the value of a figure depends on its position, or place, relative to other figures.

Look at 426. When you say the number you read it from the left – the first figure you read in a three-figure whole number is the number of hundreds, so you say 'four hundred and twenty-six'. If you didn't know how to say it you could build it up from the right: the figure furthest to the right (6) is the number of ones, the figure next to it (2) is the number of tens and the next figure (4) is the number of hundreds. Each figure is ten times larger than its neighbour to the right and ten times smaller than its neighbour to the left: this is why our number system is called a 'base ten' or decimal system.

The same principle applies with larger numbers. For example, one thousand is written 1,000 or 1 000. The zeroes are in a group of three (with a gap or a comma – in this book we use a gap because this is standard in the metric (SI) system) in order to make it easier to read. In this case, you 'read' the comma or gap as 'thousand' so 3 200 will be read as 'three thousand two hundred'.

Now look at 1 000 000 (one million). Again, the zeroes are in groups of three. This time there are two groups of three zeroes after the 1. In this case you 'read' the first gap after the 1 as 'million'.

Again, if you build it up from the right you see that there are no ones, no tens, no hundreds, no thousands, no tens of thousands, no hundreds of thousands and one million. The zeroes are 'place holders' keeping the 1 in the right position.

In the case of one million, the right place for the 1 is seven places to the left – but to the left of what?

The answer is: to the left of the *decimal point*. Normally the decimal point is not shown unless the number includes decimals (strictly speaking, 'decimal fractions') – figures to the right of the decimal point. But whether it's shown or not, the decimal point is always there in spirit, marking the boundary between figures which indicate whole numbers (to the left) and figures which mean parts of one (to the right of the decimal point).

 Connections

See *3.3 Decimals and fractions* (p. 79) for more on this.

Negative numbers

A negative number is a number with a value less than zero. Think of a cold day when the temperature drops below zero degrees Celsius (0°C) to, for example, –4°C; the –4 is a negative number, signifying the number of degrees below zero.

In fact, all numbers are either negative (below zero) or positive (above zero). Negative numbers are written with a minus sign immediately before the number and positive numbers are either written without a sign (i.e. you assume a number is positive unless a minus sign indicates otherwise) or with a plus sign, as in: +8; +1 000; +0.25, etc. Whether a number is positive or negative affects what you do when you calculate with it.

 Connections

For more on temperature, see *2.1 Monitoring vital signs* (p. 19); see *3.2 The four rules of arithmetic* (p. 69) for calculating with negative numbers.

 Activities – Working with whole numbers

Task 1

Look at the number 527. Does the 2 mean 2, 20 or 200?

Task 2

In the number 72 543 what does the 2 mean?

○ ○ ◁

Task 3

Read this number in words: 63 987.

If you're stuck, read the gap as 'thousand'. Alternatively, you can build it up from the right – say to yourself, 'seven, eighty-seven, nine hundred and eighty-seven', and so on.

Task 4

Write these numbers in words: 260 001; 8 007 639; 39 124 228.

Task 5

In your maths diary, note down any large numbers which have featured in the news recently – for example, the number of people unemployed and claiming benefit or the cost of a new hospital. Get into the habit of noting down large numbers in your maths diary and think about what they mean – don't just skip over them.

▶ **3.2   The 'four rules' of arithmetic: addition, subtraction, multiplication and division**

The 'four rules' of arithmetic – *addition, subtraction, multiplication* and *division* – are the basic operations involved in calculating with whole numbers, decimals or fractions.

 Practice tip

You don't always need to calculate accurately. Before you start any operation, decide how accurate you need to be and estimate or calculate accurately, as appropriate.

You are probably fairly familiar with all the 'four rules'; however, you may not be very confident in your ability to calculate, especially with large or awkward numbers, and you may not be aware of how the basic operations relate to each other.

How the basic operations relate to each other

Start with what you know:

- if you add or multiply (times) whole numbers you will get a result that is larger than the numbers you started with
- if you subtract (take away) or divide (share) by whole numbers the result will be smaller than the number you started with.

This gives you a clue to the relationship between addition and multiplication, and between subtraction and division, but what is the relationship?

- Multiplication is repeated addition.

For example, 3×4 means 3 times 4 (or $4 + 4 + 4$). In multiplication the order of the numbers being multiplied doesn't matter, so 3×4 is the same as 4×3 (or $3 + 3 + 3 + 3$); the answer (also known as the product) is still 12.

- Division is repeated subtraction.

For example, $15 \div 5$ means that if you start with 15 you need to take away three lots of 5 in order to get down to zero.

Factors
Factors multiply together to make another number: for example, in $8 \times 3 = 24$, 8 and 3 are factors of 24.

In $6 \times 4 = 24$, 6 and 4 are factors of 24. Similarly, in $24 \div 6 = 4$, or $24 \div 4 = 6$, you can see that the same factors are involved.

Practise breaking down numbers into factors. It will help you to see relationships between numbers in terms of multiplication and division.

Using your head
You probably already use your head to calculate but you may not feel very confident about doing so. You may feel that 'doing sums' with pen and paper is preferable to the informal methods you've worked out for yourself, even if those methods work. If so, ask yourself why you think so – after all, if your method is reliable and it works, why not use it? This is an issue you might like to explore in your maths diary.

In any case, it's a good idea to practise methods of calculating which you can do in your head – you always have your head with you whereas you can't always reach for pen and paper or a calculator.

Practice tip

- Identify the kind of operation required.
- Identify the numbers concerned.
- Break the calculation down into stages.
- Round numbers up or down to make them easier to handle.

For example, if you need to add 18 and 39, add 2 to round the 18 up to 20 and 1 to round the 39 up to 40. Add 20 and 40 to give 60, then take off the 2 to give 58 and then the 1 to give the final answer: 57.

Alternatively, you could say 18 plus 2 is 20, plus 7 is 27, plus 30 is 57.

The same approach works with subtraction as well as addition, and with large or awkward numbers – try it out in your maths diary.

You may find calculations involving multiplication a bit more tricky. However, the same principles apply, especially if the calculation involves more than one operation – for example, adding a list of numbers together and then multiplying the total by another number: break the calculation down into stages and round numbers up or down to make them easier to handle.

If you don't know your 'times tables', don't despair. Make yourself a multiplication square like the one on p. 72 on a piece of card and use it as a 'ready reckoner' for multiplication and division (e.g. for 7 × 8 just read along the line beginning with 7 and down the column beginning with 8; they intersect at the answer: 56).

The square shown is 10 × 10 but you can make yours 12 × 12, or whatever you like.

Look for patterns, for example, in the 5 times table, where the numbers end with 5 or 0 alternately – does the pattern persist beyond 10 × 5?

In the 9 times table, up to 10 × 9 the figures always add up to 9; can you see any other patterns in the 9 times table?

The 10 times table is especially easy because you just put 0 on the end of the number you want to multiply by 10; for example, 6 × 10 = 60.

This works for any whole number multiplied by 10, as you'd expect if you're clear about how place value works.

 Connections

Look at *3.1 Whole numbers* (p. 67) to remind yourself of the basic facts of place value.

A multiplication square: 10 × 10

1	2	3	4	5	6	7	8	9	10
2	4	6	8	10	12	14	16	18	20
3	6	9	12	15	18	21	24	27	30
4	8	12	16	20	24	28	32	36	40
5	10	15	20	25	30	35	40	45	50
6	12	18	24	30	36	42	48	54	60
7	14	21	28	35	42	49	56	63	70
8	16	24	32	40	48	56	64	72	80
9	18	27	36	45	54	63	72	81	90
10	20	30	40	50	60	70	80	90	100

Division

Division, especially 'long division' (dividing by a large number), may present more of a challenge. However, if you look for patterns and build on what you know, you may surprise yourself.

For example, find 72 on the multiplication square; you will see that 8 and 9 are factors of 72, so 72 is 9 × 8 (or 8 × 9). By the same token, 72 divided by 9 is 8 (72 ÷ 9 = 8) and 72 divided by 8 is 9 (72 ÷ 8 = 9).

Calculating on paper

However good you are at calculating in your head, there may still be times when you need to check your working out on paper. This is when memories of school maths lessons may come flooding back and it's easy to get hung up on trying to remember the method you were once taught, rather than using your experience and common sense.

Many people don't realise that there is more than one way of doing each of the basic operations. For example, subtraction may be done by 'counting on', by 'equal addition' (also known as the 'borrowing' method) and by 'decomposition' – all three methods are ancient and well established. Of course, you only need to use one method. Here they are:

- *Subtraction by 'counting on'*

$$64 - $$
$$38$$
$$\overline{26}$$

Look at the numbers as a whole: count on from 38 to 40 (= 2); count on from 40 to 60 (= 20); count on from 60 to 64 (= 4); add 2 and 20 and 4 (2 + 20 + 4 = 26), so the answer is 26. This method is similar to what you do in your head when giving or getting change.

- *Subtraction by 'equal addition' or 'borrowing'*

$$6^14 - $$
$$^13\ 8$$
$$\overline{2\ 6}$$

Start from the right-hand (units) column: 8 is larger than 4 so you need to borrow one lot of 10 from the next column (you show this by putting the little ^{1} next to the 4 to make 14); now take 8 away from 14 (14 – 8 = 6); write the 6 in the units column; now 'pay back' the 10 you borrowed (back in its own column it's only worth 1; show this by putting the little ^{1} next to the 3 and adding it to make 4); take 4 away from 6 (6 – 4 = 2), so the answer is 26.

- *Subtraction by 'decomposition'*

$$^56^14 - $$
$$3\ 8$$
$$\overline{2\ 6}$$

In this method you split the numbers into hundreds, tens and units ('decomposition') and reassemble them. Split 64 into 50 + 14, crossing out the 6 and replacing it with 5; take 8 away from 14 (14 – 8 = 6); take 3 away from 5 (5 – 3 = 2), so the answer is 26.

Similarly, there are several ways of writing divisions, for example:

$$15 \div 3 = 5 \quad \text{or} \quad 3\overline{)15} \quad \text{or} \quad 3)15(5 \quad \text{or} \quad \tfrac{15}{3} = 5$$

You may find it easier to write a division operation as a fraction, especially if it entails large or awkward numbers, simplifying the numbers as necessary, rather than doing a long division.

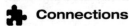 **Connections**

Turn to *3.3 Decimals and fractions* (p. 79) to refresh your memory of fractions.

If you have to do a long division, such as 1 567 divided by 23, here's how . . .

Start at the left-hand end of the number; in this case, say 'How many 23s in 156?' Use 'trial and error' multiplication to work this out – try 6 × 23 (this is a good guess because 6 × 25 = 150); 6 × 23 = 138, so write down the 6; this is the first part of your answer.

You can write the answer either above the line

$$
\begin{array}{r}
6 \\
\text{as } 23)\overline{1\ 567}
\end{array}
$$

or on the right-hand side as

$$23)\overline{1\ 567}(\,6$$

Write the 138 under the 156 to show that you are taking away:

$$
\begin{array}{r}
6 \\
23)\overline{1567} \\
138- \\
\hline
18
\end{array}
$$

Bring down the 7 to give you 187:

$$
\begin{array}{r}
6 \\
23)\overline{1567} \\
138- \\
\hline
187
\end{array}
$$

Now divide 187 by 23 using 'trial and error' multiplication again: try 7 × 23 which comes to 161, so you can probably see that another 23 would bring it up to 184. In other words, 8 × 23 = 184, so write the 8 next to the 6, to give you the answer, 68.

$$
\begin{array}{r}
68 \\
23\overline{)1567} \\
138- \\
\hline
187 \\
184- \\
\hline
3
\end{array}
$$

Take 184 away from 187, leaving you with a remainder, 3.

What do you do with the remainder?
There are at least three ways of handling any remainder; which you use will depend on the context and how accurate you need to be:

- you can write 'remainder 3'
- you can put the 3 over the number you're dividing by (the 23) to express the remainder as a fraction ($\frac{3}{23}$)
- you can put a decimal point followed by a zero after the last figure in the number you're dividing into (1 567.0) and continue dividing (putting in more zeroes to signify decimal places as necessary).

Calculating with a calculator
Correctly used, a calculator enables you to calculate accurately and frees you to experiment with calculations and estimate the correct answer as a checking mechanism.

Calculators vary (for example, the sign for multiply may be x or *, and the sign for divide may be ÷ or /), but with most, you simply press the keys in the order in which you say the numbers to yourself as you perform the operation (this is known as the 'key sequence').

For example, with addition, if you press ⬚3 ⬚4 ⬚+ ⬚5 ⬚6 ⬚= in the order they're written here, you'll get the correct answer: 90. Similarly, with subtraction, ⬚2 ⬚5 ⬚- ⬚1 ⬚6 ⬚= will give you the answer 9; with multiplication, ⬚7 ⬚6 ⬚× ⬚2 ⬚= will give you the answer 152; with division, ⬚5 ⬚5 ⬚÷ ⬚1 ⬚1 ⬚= will give you the answer 5 (but be careful to key in '55 divided by 11' rather than '11 into 55' – see *The order of operations*, p. 76).

It's a good idea to estimate the answer first – that way you're more likely to notice if you key in the wrong number or if you don't press the decimal-point button correctly. You need to have an idea of the size of the numbers you're dealing with, as an error made with a calculator can result in an overdose or underdose in the order of 10, 100 or 1000 times, or more.

Also, if you press the C (Clear) key, or turn the calculator off and on again between operations, you won't accidentally 'run on' numbers from one calculation to the next. Check your answer by repeating the calculation on your calculator or by doing it in your head or on paper. Get to know your calculator and have fun!

The order of operations

What if you need to do a calculation which involves more than one operation – does it matter which order you do it in?

If the operations concerned are addition and subtraction then it doesn't matter what the order is; you'll still get the same answer, as this example shows: 6 + 3 – 4 – 2 = 3 and –4 + 3 + 6 – 2 = 3 (look at *negative numbers*, in *3.1 Whole numbers* (p. 67), if this isn't clear).

For convenience, we usually set out a subtraction calculation so that the smaller number is clearly taken away from the larger number, e.g. you'd write 16 – 3, rather than –3 +16, but the order doesn't affect the outcome since the sign immediately before the number indicates whether the number is behaving as a positive or negative number and, in effect, tells you whether to add or subtract it.

Similarly, the order doesn't matter if the operation concerned is multiplication, as we have seen: 3 × 5 = 15 and 5 × 3 = 15 also.

The order *does* matter if the calculation involves division, since, for example, 8 ÷ 2 = 4 but 2 ÷ 8 = 0.25. You can usually tell from the context which number to divide by which, for example, 20ml of medicine in four equal doses is 20 ÷ 4 = 5ml; you're unlikely to try and divide 4 by 20 if you relate the calculation to the context.

The order *does* matter, also, if the calculation involves multiplication or division as well as addition and subtraction. For example, you might think that 2 + 4 × 3 – 8 meant 'add 2 and 4 together and then multiply the product, 6, by 3 and finally take away 8'; this would give you the answer 10. But if you do the multiplication first you get the answer 6, as: 4 times 3 is 12, plus 2 is 14, minus 8 is 6.

So how do you know which order is correct?

If there are brackets in the calculation, always do the operations in brackets first, so, for example, –(9 + 3) = –12.

However, if there is no indication in the form of brackets and you can't tell from the context where they should be, the rule is to deal with any multiplication or division first, before moving on to any addition or subtraction. In the example above, this would give you (4 × 3) + 2 – 8, which works out as 12 + 2 – 8 = 6.

If you come across sets of brackets next to each other with no signs in between, this means you should multiply the products of the brackets together, as in: $(5 + 4)(6 - 3) = 9 \times 3 = 27$.

Indices

You will come across index numbers (plural: indices), for example, in association with metric measurements in laboratory reports. Indices are used to minimise the risk of mistakes caused by miscounting zeroes in very large or very small numbers.

Indices are also known as 'powers'. The index figure tells you how many times a number has been multiplied by itself. For example, $2 \times 2 \times 2 \times 2$ is 2^4, which you'd say as '2 to the power of 4'.

You can compare numbers expressed in this way without doing any multiplication, providing the base number is the same. In this case, for example, the base number is 2 and 2^4 is bigger than 2^3 (try multiplying it if you're not convinced).

For powers of 10 the rules are:

- For numbers greater than one, the index figure is the same as the number of zeroes. For example, one thousand (1 000) is 10^3; this is because $1\,000 = 1 \times 10 \times 10 \times 10$ and the little ^{3} tells you how many times ten has been multiplied by itself to give 1 000; 10^3 is '10 to the power of 3'.
- For numbers less than one, the index number has a minus sign and indicates the decimal place of the first figure (other than zero) to the right of the decimal point. For example, one microgram is 0.000 001 gram, which would be written as 10^{-6}g with the little ^{6} indicating that the figure 1 is in the sixth decimal place (meaning $1 \div 10 \div 10 \div 10 \div 10 \div 10 \div 10$); you'd say '10 to the power of minus 6'.

 Connection

For help with decimals, turn to *3.3 Decimals and fractions* (p. 79).

Standard form

Armed with this knowledge, you can express any number in what's known as 'standard form', making it easier to compare the size of numbers. For example, 2 000 is 2×10^3; 500 is 5×10^2; and so on. In this case it's obvious that 2 000 is bigger than 500, but if you are dealing with a very large or very small number where the difference isn't obvious, this method enables you to compare relative sizes by comparing the powers of 10: the larger the index figure, the larger the number.

This works for any whole number: just rewrite the number as a decimal with one whole number (i.e. in the case of 2 000, rewrite it as 2.000) and then multiply by the appropriate power of 10 (in this case, 10^3; you work out what the index is by counting the number of decimal places in 2.000, including the zeroes, to give you 2.000×10^3 or 2×10^3). Try it with more complicated numbers – like 365 or 49 630 – until you're comfortable using standard form.

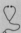

Practice tip

- Remember the rules of place value (see *3.1 Whole numbers* (p. 67)).
- Choose a method which suits you and the circumstances best and decide whether you need to estimate or calculate accurately.
- Estimate first when calculating accurately, especially when using a calculator.
- Check your answer by using another method (on paper, in your head or using a calculator).
- If you get stuck, try the same operation but with easier numbers.
- If you know the answer but can't see how to get there, work backwards from the answer to reconstruct the stages in the calculation.
- Relate the calculation to the context – always remember what it is you're trying to find out.
- Make a note of tricky operations in your maths diary and practise to extend the limits of your calculating ability.

Activities – Working with the 'four rules'

Task 1

Add 3 099 and 408 and 2 122 in your head, on paper and with a calculator.

Task 2

Divide 360 by 9 in your head.

Task 3

Multiply 48 by 100 in your head.

○ ○ ▷

Task 4

Subtract 650 from 4 789 and multiply the result by 6.

Task 5

$(76 + 450) - (240 \div 8) =$ _____

Task 6

Express 7 830 in standard form.

Task 7

Express 10^{-5} as a decimal.

Task 8

Arrange these numbers in size order with the largest number first:
4^6; 4^8; 4^3; 4^2

▶ **3.3 Decimals and fractions**

Decimals and fractions are two different ways of representing parts of a
whole.

Decimals

Decimals (strictly speaking 'decimal fractions') are written as figures to
the right of the decimal point, like pence in a sum of money.

Start with what you know. Look at, for example, £1.57. You know that
57p is five 10 pence and 7 pence. The 5 is immediately to the right of the
decimal point because in that position it tells you how many 10 pence
there are.

Decimals are all about the position of figures in relation to the decimal
point. Knowing what decimals are is the first step towards being able to
recognise and use them with confidence.

Look back at £1.57. You know that the 5 means the number of 10
pence. You know also that there are ten 10p in £1. Each 10p is worth one-
tenth of £1, so here you're dealing with five-tenths of £1. There are seven
single pence, each one of which is worth one-hundredth of £1, because
100p make £1.

In a sum of money, the decimal point separates the pounds (on the left)
from the pence (on the right), or the whole pounds from the parts of a
pound. It's the same for a number that isn't a sum of money: the decimal

point separates the whole numbers (on the left) from the parts of one (on the right).

For example, suppose a patient's temperature is 36.8°C, what does this mean? The patient's temperature is 36 whole degrees Celsius plus .8 ('point 8') of a degree. In other words, it's well over 36 degrees but not quite 37 degrees.

Clinical mercury thermometers normally show only one decimal place. In a sum of money you only have two decimal places: in £1.57, five 10 pence and seven pence. In a number that isn't a sum of money or a temperature there may be more than two figures to the right of the decimal point.

Rounding off decimals
You don't always need to be exact. In circumstances where an approximate figure is adequate, you can *round off* the decimals to an appropriate number of decimal places.

For example, suppose you need to round off 4.73 ('four point seven three') to one decimal place.

Look at the number as a whole and think what it means: 4.73 means four whole ones, seven-tenths and three-hundredths (or four whole ones and 73-hundredths). You can probably see that it's closer to 4.7 than 4.8.

Now look at each figure in turn, starting with the figure furthest to the right, the 3 (meaning 3-hundredths). The rule is, if the figure on the right is less than 5 then the figure next to it on the left stays the same; if it's 5 or more than 5, then the figure next to it goes up one. In this case, 3 is less than 5, so the 7 stays as it is. So 4.73 is 4.7 correct to one decimal place.

Calculating with decimals in your head
One way of making calculations with decimals easier is to round them off. Some people visualise the sum written down and work through it in their mind's eye, using their fingers if necessary, and some lucky people just *see* the answer. Even if you prefer to calculate with decimals on paper or with a calculator, it's still a good idea to estimate the answer first.

Calculating with decimals on paper
Adding. Line up the figures so that the decimal points are directly underneath each other – this is important to ensure that you add tenths to tenths and hundredths to hundredths.

You can fill in blanks with zeroes as place holders so long as they are not placed between the decimal point and another number – for example, 0.6 is the same as 0.60 and .78 is the same as 0.78.

Add the figures column by column, starting from the right.

```
0.78 +          0.6 +
0.24            3.27
----            ----
1.02            3.87
```

Subtracting
Again, line up the figures so that the decimal points are directly under-neath each other with the larger number on top (remember to look at the number as a whole when deciding which is larger, not just the decimals).

You can put the minus sign either on the left or the right, and next to either figure:

```
3.57 –              3.57
1.63              – 1.63
----              ------
1.94                1.94
```

Multiplying
It doesn't matter which number you multiply by which, since you'll get the same answer either way. You can put the multiplication sign either on the left or the right and next to either number and you can start multiplying from the left- or right-hand end:

```
 starting with 9            starting with 6
    52.1 ×                     52.1
    6.9                      × 6.9
    ----                     ------
    4689                     31260
   31260                      4689
  -------                    -------
   359.49                     359.49
```

When multiplying decimals, ignore the decimal point until the end, when you count how many decimals there are altogether in the two numbers you multiplied together.

You then count that number of decimal places in from the right of your answer and put the decimal point in at that position.

There are two figures after the decimal point (9 and 1) in 6.9 and 52.1, so count two decimal places in from the right and put the decimal point there. The answer is 359.49.

Dividing
Dividing a decimal by a whole number is quite straightforward. Just work your way through, dividing each number in turn, for example, $8.64 \div 2 = 4.32$.

To divide a decimal by a decimal, for example, 78.36 ÷ 1.2, convert the number you're dividing by (in this case 1.2) into a whole number by multiplying it by 10 or a multiple of 10 in order to get rid of the decimal point; this gives you 12.

Do the same to the number you're dividing into (in this case multiply 78.36 by 10) in order to keep the same relative values; this gives 783.6.

Then continue with the division: 783.6 ÷ 12.

You can write this out as a long division:

```
        65.3
12)783.6
    72
    ──
    63
    60
    ──
    36
```

The answer is 65.3.

Since you've kept the proportions the same by multiplying both 783.6 and 1.2 by 10, you don't adjust the answer – if 783.6 ÷ 12 = 65.3, so does 78.36 ÷ 1.2 = 65.3. Check this with a calculator if you're sceptical.

Calculating with decimals using a calculator
Key in each figure and sign in turn, being careful to key in the decimal point in the correct position. It's a good idea to estimate the answer in your head first so that you'll notice if you press the wrong keys and get a wrong answer.

 Connections

If this isn't clear, check *3.2 The four rules of arithmetic* (p. 69).

Fractions

Fractions like a half ($\frac{1}{2}$) or a quarter ($\frac{1}{4}$) (otherwise picturesquely known as 'vulgar' or 'common' fractions) are another means of expressing parts of a whole.

Sometimes you may find it easier to use decimals (decimal fractions) like 0.5 or 0.25 and sometimes 'ordinary' fractions (vulgar fractions). Use whichever suits you – and the circumstances – best.

If you are using fractions, start with what you know:

two halves make a whole one: $2 \times \frac{1}{2} = 1$

four quarters make a whole one: $4 \times \frac{1}{4} = 1$

Fractions are written with one number over another in order to indicate the relationship between them.

The number at the bottom (called the 'denominator') tells you (or 'denominates') how many parts the whole has been split into.

The number at the top (the numerator) tells you how many parts you're dealing with in this instance.

For example, $\frac{1}{3}$ means that a whole one is divided into three equal parts and you're dealing with one part; $\frac{2}{3}$ means that you're dealing with two of the parts.

The line separating the top and bottom numbers of a fraction is another way of saying 'divide', for example:

a half is one divided by two $1 \div 2 = \frac{1}{2}$

a quarter is one divided by four $1 \div 4 = \frac{1}{4}$

Simplifying fractions
Simplifying fractions (also known as 'cancelling') makes them more user-friendly – it doesn't alter the meaning or value of the fraction because the relationship between the top and bottom numbers is maintained.

To simplify fractions, divide the top and bottom numbers by the same number.

For example, $\frac{7}{21}$ can be rewritten as $\frac{1}{3}$ because you can divide both top and bottom numbers by the same number (7), which gives you $\frac{1}{3}$.

Calculating with fractions
You can avoid calculating with fractions by converting fractions into decimals and calculating with decimals instead – see *Converting fractions to decimals*, p. 86.

Adding fractions
WHEN THE BOTTOM NUMBERS (THE DENOMINATORS) ARE THE SAME
You're adding like to like – just add the top numbers, leaving the bottom number as it is.

For example,

$$\frac{1}{4} + \frac{1}{4} = \frac{1}{2}$$

WHEN THE BOTTOM NUMBERS (THE DENOMINATORS) ARE DIFFERENT

Change one or both fractions so that the bottom numbers are the same (known as 'the common denominator'). You find this by working out the lowest number that both the original denominators can be divided into.

For example, in the sum $\frac{1}{4} + \frac{2}{3}$ the lowest number that both 4 and 3 can be divided into is 12, so 12 is the common denominator.

Once you've found the common denominator, look at each fraction in turn and express it in terms of the common denominator (this is rather like simplifying the fraction in reverse).

In this case, 12 ÷ 4 is 3, and 3 x 1 = 3, therefore $\frac{1}{4} = \frac{3}{12}$.

Similarly, 12 divided by 3 is 4, and 4 times 2 is 8, therefore $\frac{2}{3} = \frac{8}{12}$.

Once you've expressed both the original fractions in terms of their common denominator, in this case $\frac{3}{12} + \frac{8}{12}$, just add the top numbers together and leave the bottom number as it is, 3 + 8 = 11, so the answer is $\frac{11}{12}$.

Subtracting fractions

Subtracting fractions works in the same way, but unless you're dealing with negative numbers you must be sure to subtract the smaller fraction from the larger. If you're not sure which is the larger in the original, simplify the fractions as far as possible and then find their common denominator – it should be obvious which is larger by then as you will be comparing like with like, for example, $\frac{8}{12}$ is larger than $\frac{3}{12}$ because there are more twelfths in $\frac{8}{12}$ than there are in $\frac{3}{12}$.

Here is an example of a subtraction with fractions:

$$\frac{7}{21} - \frac{3}{12}$$

The first step is to simplify the fractions by cancelling:

$$\frac{7}{21} - \frac{3}{12} = \frac{1}{3} - \frac{1}{4}$$

Then turn the fractions into the same type of fraction (fractions with the same denominator). The lowest number that both 4 and 3 can be divided into is 12, so 12 is the common denominator.

You already know that $\frac{1}{4}$ equals $\frac{3}{12}$.

You can work out that $\frac{1}{3}$ equals $\frac{4}{12}$ because there are 4 lots of 3 in 12, therefore each $\frac{1}{3}$ equals $\frac{4}{12}$.

So: $\frac{7}{21} - \frac{3}{12} = \frac{1}{3} - \frac{1}{4} = \frac{4}{12} - \frac{3}{12} = \frac{1}{12}$.

Multiplying a fraction by a fraction
As you see from an easy example, $\frac{1}{2} \times \frac{1}{2} = \frac{1}{4}$, all you do to multiply a fraction by a fraction is to multiply the top number by the top number and the bottom number by the bottom number and then simplify the resulting fraction if necessary.

Remember that 'x' means 'of', so $\frac{1}{2} \times \frac{1}{2}$ means 'half of a half'.

Multiplying a fraction by a whole number
Again, an easy example gives you the clue: $2 \times \frac{1}{2} = 1$.

A whole number can be written over 1 (because dividing by 1 leaves the number unchanged), so $2 = \frac{2}{1}$.

Rewrite the fraction calculation as $\frac{2}{1} \times \frac{1}{2}$, then proceed as when multiplying a fraction by a fraction: multiply the top number by the top number and the bottom number by the bottom number and then simplify the resulting fraction, if necessary.

In the example, $2 \times 1 = 2$ and $1 \times 2 = 2$, giving you $\frac{2}{2}$, which simplifies to give the answer: 1.

Dividing a fraction by a fraction
To divide a fraction by a fraction, for example, $\frac{2}{3} \div \frac{1}{4}$, first change the $\div$ to x and turn the $\frac{1}{4}$ upside down: $\frac{4}{1}$, giving you $\frac{2}{3} \times \frac{4}{1}$.

Then proceed as when multiplying a fraction by a fraction. This may sound like a trick but try it and see!

It may help to remember that $\frac{1}{2}$ is another way of saying 1 divided by 2; in other words, when you multiply something by $\frac{1}{2}$ you are halving it – or dividing it by two.

Mixed fractions
A mixed fraction, for example, $2\frac{1}{3}$, is a whole number and a fraction.

You can express a mixed fraction as an improper fraction (meaning that the numerator is larger than the denominator).

To do this, multiply the whole number by the denominator ($2 \times 3 = 6$) and add the numerator ($6 + 1 = 7$), so $2\frac{1}{3} = \frac{7}{3}$.

Once you've turned the mixed fraction into an improper fraction you can calculate with it just as with any other fraction.

Converting fractions to decimals and vice versa

Converting decimals to fractions

Look back at *Decimals* on p. 79. Decimals are another way of expressing tenths, hundredths, thousandths, etc.; decimals and fractions can be expressed in equivalent terms.

For example, $0.5 = \frac{5}{10}$ which simplifies to $\frac{1}{2}$; in other words, $0.5 = \frac{1}{2}$.

Similarly, $0.25 = \frac{25}{100}$ which simplifies to $\frac{1}{4}$, so $0.25 = \frac{1}{4}$.

In other words, any single figure decimal can be expressed as tenths, any double figure decimal can be expressed as hundredths, and so on.

Converting fractions to decimals

Suppose you want to convert a fraction that isn't tenths, hundredths, etc. to a decimal – what do you do then?

Well, suppose you want to convert $\frac{2}{5}$ to a decimal.

Start with what you know: a fraction is another way of expressing the division of the top number by the bottom number.

$\frac{2}{5}$ is another way of saying 2 divided by 5.

You can write this as

$5\overline{)2}$

Say '5 into 2 won't go, put down 0'; 0 is the first part of your answer.

Then put a decimal point followed by 0 after the 2, giving you $5\overline{)2.0}^{\,0}$ and say '5 into 20 goes 4'.

Put down the 4 after the 0 in your answer, $5\overline{)2.0}^{\,0.4}$ with a decimal point between the 0 and the 4. This gives you the answer, 0.4.

Practise this with different fractions.

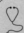
Practice tip

Tips for calculating with decimals and fractions:

- Decide whether to use decimals or fractions in a particular operation.
- Choose a calculating method (in your head; on paper; with a calculator) which suits you and the circumstances best.
- Estimate first by rounding off awkward numbers.
- Check your answer by using another method (on paper, in your head or using a calculator).
- Make a note of situations in which you encounter decimals and fractions in your maths diary and practise to extend the limits of your calculating ability.
- If calculating with fractions is a headache, first convert your fractions to decimals and then do the calculation.
- It's not always easy to compare the size of fractions (for example, deciding whether $\frac{2}{5}$ is bigger than $\frac{3}{7}$). Try converting them to decimals.

Activities – Working with decimals and fractions

Task 1

Express 0.01 as a fraction.

Task 2

Convert $\frac{7}{20}$ to a decimal.

Task 3

$0.25 \times 3.64 = $ _____

Task 4

$\frac{42.5}{25} = $ _____

Task 5

$0.008\ 1 \div 0.9 = $ _____

Task 6

$\frac{75}{100} + \frac{20}{80} = $ _____

Task 7

Simplify these fractions: $\frac{16}{32}$; $\frac{50}{200}$; $\frac{25}{150}$; $\frac{36}{540}$.

▶ 3.4   Percentages

Per cent means 'out of every hundred'; it's written %. For example, 50% means 50 out of every hundred – in other words, half. Percentages make it easier to see patterns and to deal with relationships between awkward numbers.

What if you want to find a percentage of a number, for example, 10% of 30? You can work this out in your head, or on paper, or you can use a calculator.

In your head
Look at 10% of 30 and work from there. You know that 10% is one-tenth, so 10% of 30 is 3.

This is because to find 10% all you need to do is divide the number in question (in this case 30) by 10. The answer is 3; because 30 divided by 10 gives you the answer 3.

On paper
10% can be written as a fraction: $\frac{10}{100}$.

$\frac{10}{100}$ can be simplified to $\frac{1}{10}$.

Just divide the top part of $\frac{10}{100}$ by 10 and then do the same to the bottom part.

'Of' can be written as **×** meaning multiply or 'times'.

One tenth of 30 means $\frac{1}{10} \times 30$ or 30 divided by 10, so the answer is 3.

With a calculator
If your calculator has a % key, press either $\boxed{1}$ $\boxed{0}$ $\boxed{\times}$ $\boxed{3}$ $\boxed{0}$ $\boxed{\%}$ or $\boxed{3}$ $\boxed{0}$ $\boxed{\times}$ $\boxed{1}$ $\boxed{0}$ $\boxed{\%}$.

On some calculators you have to press $\boxed{=}$ after $\boxed{\%}$; on others you just press $\boxed{\%}$.

If there is no $\boxed{\%}$ key, press *either* $\boxed{1}$ $\boxed{0}$ $\boxed{\div}$ $\boxed{1}$ $\boxed{0}$ $\boxed{0}$ $\boxed{\times}$ $\boxed{3}$ $\boxed{0}$ $\boxed{=}$ *or* $\boxed{1}$ $\boxed{0}$ $\boxed{/}$ $\boxed{1}$ $\boxed{0}$ $\boxed{0}$ $\boxed{*}$ $\boxed{3}$ $\boxed{0}$ $\boxed{=}$.

Whichever way you choose, the answer is 3.

Similarly, if you wanted to find 40% of 280, you could work it out in your head, or on paper, or you could use a calculator.

In your head
Look at 40% of 280 and work from there.

Break down 40% into 4 lots of 10%.
Work out 10% of 280.

10% of 280 is 28. This is because to find 10% all you need to do is divide the number in question (in this case 280) by 10.

Check this on paper or with a calculator if it isn't obvious.

Now work out 4 times 28; you may find it easier to do this in stages:
$28 + 28 = 56$; $56 + 56 = 112$.

On paper
40% of 280.

40% can be written as a fraction: $\frac{40}{100}$.

'Of' can be written as x meaning multiply or 'times', so

either
$\frac{40}{100} \times 280 = \frac{2}{5} \times 280 = 112$

or
$\frac{40}{100} \times 280 = \frac{40}{10} \times 28 = \frac{4}{1} \times 28 = 112$.

With a calculator
If your calculator has a $\boxed{\%}$ key, press either $\boxed{4}$ $\boxed{0}$ $\boxed{\times}$ $\boxed{2}$ $\boxed{8}$ $\boxed{0}$ $\boxed{\%}$
or $\boxed{2}$ $\boxed{8}$ $\boxed{0}$ $\boxed{\times}$ $\boxed{4}$ $\boxed{0}$ $\boxed{\%}$.

If there is no $\boxed{\%}$ key, press *either* $\boxed{4}$ $\boxed{0}$ $\boxed{\div}$ $\boxed{1}$ $\boxed{0}$ $\boxed{0}$ $\boxed{\times}$ $\boxed{2}$ $\boxed{8}$
$\boxed{0}$ $\boxed{=}$ *or* $\boxed{4}$ $\boxed{0}$ $\boxed{/}$ $\boxed{1}$ $\boxed{0}$ $\boxed{0}$ $\boxed{*}$ $\boxed{2}$ $\boxed{8}$ $\boxed{0}$ $\boxed{=}$.

To express one number as a percentage of another
What if you need to express one number as a percentage of another?

Imagine you are dealing with a population of 20 000 people and you know that 5 000 of them are over 60 years old. You want to know what proportion of the whole population is over 60. You can do this by expressing the two population figures in percentage terms.

To express one number as a percentage of another, think of what it is you want to know. In this case, you want to know the percentage of over-60s in the whole population. You might find it easier to think of this as 'what fraction of the population is over 60?'

Well, it's 5 000 out of 20 000, or 5 000 twenty-thousandths, or $\frac{5\,000}{20\,000}$.

This is an awkward fraction, but you can make it more user-friendly.

To begin with, you could simplify it by 'cancelling out' the zeroes, giving you $\frac{5\,000}{20\,000} = \frac{5}{20}$.

Next you could divide the top and bottom numbers by something (*providing it's the same something*). In this case 5 divides into 5 and 20 exactly, so the user-friendly version of $\frac{5\,000}{20\,000}$ is $\frac{5}{20}$ or $\frac{1}{4}$.

In other words, a quarter of the population is over 60, but what is that as a percentage?

You may already know that $\frac{1}{4}$ is 25%, or you can work it out in stages:

a quarter of the whole population is over 60
the whole population is 100%
a quarter of 100 is 25
so a quarter is 25%
25% of the population is over 60.

Most of the time the numbers don't work out so neatly, so you'll need to look back at what you've just done: $\frac{5\,000}{20\,000}$.

If you can't see a way to make it more user-friendly, number-crunch it.

Remember that $\frac{5\,000}{20\,000}$ also means 5 000 ÷ 20 000 (because the dividing line in a fraction between the top and bottom numbers is just that – a *dividing* line: it means 'divide the top number by the bottom number').

Try that on a calculator and you'll get 0.25. So 0.25 of the population is over 60. What does that mean in percentage terms?

Well, 0.25 means 25-hundredths, 25-hundredths means 25 out of 100, and that's another way of saying 25%.

Once you've got your answer as a decimal you can read it off as a percentage: 0.25 = 25%.

You can also work out 5 000 as a percentage of 20 000 in your head, or on paper, or you can use a calculator.

In your head
Look at 5 000 and 20 000 and work from there.

Start with what you know: you know that 20 000 is the whole population (i.e. 100%) for the purposes of this calculation.

Break the calculation down into easy stages: if 100% is 20 000, 50% must be 10 000, so half of 10 000 will give you 5 000, which must be 25%

On paper (fraction method)

Multiply $\frac{5\,000}{20\,000}$ by 100 to turn it into a percentage:

$\frac{5\,000}{20\,000} \times 100 = \frac{5}{20} \times 100 = \frac{1}{4} \times 100 = 25.$

With a calculator

Press *either* [5] [0] [0] [0] [÷] [2] [0] [0] [0] [0] [×] [1] [0] [0] [=]

or [5] [0] [0] [0] [/] [2] [0] [0] [0] [0] [*] [1] [0] [0] [=].

Whichever method you choose, the answer is 25%.
In other words, 25% of the given population is over 60.

Use the method which suits you – and the circumstances – best.

 Practice tip

Tips for calculating with percentages

- Identify what you want to use percentages for: what do you want to find out?
- Choose a calculating method (in your head; on paper; with a calculator) which suits you and the circumstances best.
- Estimate first by rounding off awkward numbers.
- Check your answer by using another method (on paper, in your head or using a calculator).
- Make a note of situations in which you encounter percentages in your maths diary and practise to extend the limits of your calculating ability.

 Activities – Working with percentages

Task 1

What is: 50% of 600?
        15% of 4 500?

Task 2

How many litres of dextrose are contained in 3 litres of 10% dextrose?

Task 3

Express 500 as a percentage of 25 000; 200 as a percentage of 8 000.

Task 4

The incidence of heart disease in a given population is 2%. If the total population is 150 000, how many people have heart disease?

▶ 3.5   Ratios

Ratios are used in many different situations in healthcare, for example, to express the strength of a drug in solution, or the incidence of a disease or disorder, or the number of nurses in relation to the number of patients.

Let's start by looking at an example involving a drug diluted in a stock solution.

A dilution of 1:5 ('one to five') means 1 part of stock solution to 5 parts of diluent (the name for any substance that dilutes or dissolves). In other words, to make the solution up to the required strength, you add 1 part of the stock solution to every 5 parts of the diluent.

The same dilution may be expressed as 1 in 6. But why?

Think of 1:5 again and add the terms together: $1 + 5 = 6$.

In other words, there are 6 parts altogether, 5 of which are diluent and 1 of which is the stock solution. There is therefore 1 part of the stock solution in every 6 parts of the total solution.

In other words, 1:5 means the same as 1 in 6.

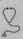   **Practice tip**

It is important not to confuse the two forms (for example, 1:6 and 1 in 6), as they will give different results, as you'll see from these examples:

How much stock solution is there in 210ml of diluted solution if the strength of the solution is 1:6?

1:6 means 1 part stock solution to every 6 parts of diluent. In other words, the total diluted solution has $6 + 1 = 7$ parts. Divide the amount of diluted solution by 7 to find how many ml there are in each part: $210 \div 7 = 30$, so there are 30ml in each part. Then look at how many parts of stock solution you are dealing with – here it is only one part, so the answer is 30ml of stock solution in 210ml of diluted solution.

IIII▶

How much stock solution is there in 210ml of diluted solution if the strength of the solution is 1 in 6?

1 in 6 means 1 part in every 6 parts of the total diluted solution is stock solution. Divide the amount of diluted solution by 6 to find how many ml there are in each part: 210 ÷ 6 = 35, so there are 35ml in each part. Then look at how many parts of stock solution you are dealing with. It is only one part, so the answer is 35ml.

As you see, the difference between the two results is 5ml, a potentially significant difference.

Not all ratios involve such straightforward calculations. If you're dealing with a ratio involving large numbers (such as 60:100) you can simplify matters by rewriting the ratio. You do this by dividing both parts of the ratio by the same number (just like simplifying a fraction and for the same reason – you're maintaining the relationship between the parts); for example, you could divide both 60 and 100 by 10, to get a ratio of 6:10 and then divide both 6 and 10 by 2 to get a ratio of 3:5, which is rather easier to handle.

Let's look at a ratio in another healthcare situation: the number of nurses in relation to the number of patients. Suppose that a ward that has been staffed by four nurses on each shift is to be reduced to two qualified nurses and three healthcare assistants. At the same time the number of patients is to be increased from 20 to 24. The previous ratio of qualified nurses to patients was 4:20; the new ratio will be 2:24. If you rewrite those ratios using the technique of dividing by the same number, you find that the ratio has gone from 1:5 to 1:12. Rewriting the ratios in this way makes it easier to compare the two situations and understand what's going on – at least in relation to the staffing levels – there may of course be other variables affecting the situation.

 Connections

See *2.7 Budget calculations* (p. 53) for more on staffing calculations.

Activities – Working with ratios

Task 1

Make a note in your maths diary of any ratios that you encounter.

Task 2

Rewrite these ratios in a more user-friendly form: 5:100; 6:12; 25:50.

Task 3

Which of these ratios mean the same?
25:100; 1:4; 2:8; 5:20; 8:24

Task 4

How much stock solution is there in 600ml of diluted solution if the strength of the solution is 1:5?

▶ 3.6 The metric (SI) system

The metric system of SI units (so-called after the International System of Units – *Système International d'Unités*) was adopted by the National Health Service in 1975 to replace the mixture of imperial, metric and apothecaries' units previously used.

We shall concentrate on some of the metric measurements most frequently encountered in healthcare:

metre (length) abbreviated to m
gram (weight or mass) abbreviated to g
litre (capacity or volume) abbreviated to L (or l or ℓ)
joule (energy) abbreviated to J
mole (molecular weight) abbreviated to mol

Practice tip

The use of capital L for litre is a printing convention throughout the *British National Formulary* – hence its use in this book. Both L and l (also written ℓ) are recognised abbreviations for SI units of capacity.

‖▶

The metric (SI) system is a decimal or base-ten system, like the number system generally (see *3.1 Whole numbers*, p. 67). Each SI unit may be combined with a prefix to indicate amounts ten – or multiples of ten times – larger and smaller than the unit.

In healthcare, the prefixes you will encounter most frequently are mega, kilo, milli and micro:

mega means one million (1 000 000) units (M)

kilo means one thousand (1 000) units (k)

milli means one thousandth ($\frac{1}{1000}$ or 0.001) of a unit (m)

micro means one millionth ($\frac{1}{1000000}$ or 0.000 001) of a unit

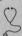

Practice tip

You may come across micro abbreviated to μ (mu, pronounced 'mew'). NEVER abbreviate micro; ALWAYS write the micro unit in full to avoid confusion with m (for milli), which is 1 000 times bigger.

Similarly, to avoid confusion, the word 'units' should not be abbreviated.

The *British National Formulary* has ruled that drug doses should be prescribed in micrograms and not as decimal parts of a milligram, but this is not always done – so BE CAREFUL!

Where decimals are unavoidable, a zero should be written in front of the decimal point where there is no other figure, for example, write 0.5ml not .5 ml.

For example:
one thousand metres (1 000m) is 1 kilometre (1km)
one thousand grams (1 000g) is 1 kilogram (1kg)
one thousand litres (1 000L) is 1 kilolitre (1kL)

one thousandth of a metre is 1 millimetre (1mm)
one thousandth of a gram is 1 milligram (1mg)
one thousandth of a litre is 1 millilitre (1ml)

one millionth of a metre (or one thousandth of a millimetre)
is 1 micrometre (DON'T abbreviate)
one millionth of a gram (or one thousandth of a milligram)
is 1 microgram (DON'T abbreviate)
one millionth of a litre (or one thousandth of a millilitre)
is 1 microlitre (DON'T abbreviate)

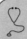 **Practice tip**

NOTE: DON'T add an 's' to abbreviated forms in the plural, for example, 5 milligrams is abbreviated to 5mg (NOT 5mgs).

Measuring weight or mass

You need to become familiar with the very small quantities involved, for example, in drug dosages as well as with larger quantities, for example, when weighing an adult patient.

Medicines to be administered in tablet form are usually listed as a given weight per tablet, such as paracetamol 500mg (see *2.6 Giving medication*, p. 45).

An adult's weight would be expressed in kilograms, while an infant's weight would be expressed in grams (see *2.2 Measuring weight and height* and *2.5 Infant feeding*, p. 43).

Measuring liquid volume

The litre is used as the standard for liquid volume and concentrations of active agents are listed as grams per litre (g/L), milligrams per millilitre (mg/ml) or as millimoles per litre (mmol/L, see below).

You may come across prescriptions using the term cc (cubic centimetre), despite the best efforts of the *British National Formulary* which has outlawed the practice. If so, you can safely assume that 1cc = 1ml because 1 litre (1 000ml) of water occupies a volume of almost exactly 1 000 cubic centimetres.

Moles

Moles measure the weight (or mass) of molecules. Molecular weights allow comparisons to be made between the weights of different compounds. Molecular weights are based on the Periodic Table which details the weights (or mass) of atoms. Since atoms combine to form molecules, atomic weights are added together to give molecular weights. A mole has a mass equal to its molecular weight expressed in grams, for example, the molecular weight of dextrose is 180, so a mole of dextrose will be 180g.

Millimoles per litre (mmol/L)

You will also come across substances in solution given as a number of millimoles per litre, abbreviated to mmol/L (see *2.3 The fluid balance chart*, p. 34).

One millimole (1 mmol) is one thousandth of a mole.

Activities – Working with the metric system

(We've given you a little help with the first task)

Task 1

Express 3g as mg.

Keep a sense of proportion. Milligrams are much smaller than grams; in fact they're 1 000 times smaller, so for any given amount of grams, you'll have 1 000 times more milligrams, so you need to multiply the 3 by 1 000.

Task 2

Express 600ml as L.

Task 3

Fill in the blanks:

400ml = ____ L
0.5g = ____ mg
0.1L = ____ ml
8 000mg = ____ g

Task 4

Write these in full:

59mg
74mmol/L
3Mg
4mJ

Task 5

Which is bigger?

1 000ml or 1L
35mg or 35g
2ml or 200L

Task 6

In your maths diary, make a note of any aspects of the metric system which you find difficult, together with a plan of action for overcoming those difficulties.

▶ 3.7 The 24-hour clock

The 24-hour clock is used on charts and timetables for conciseness and to avoid confusion between morning (a.m.) and afternoon and evening (p.m.) times.

Times in the morning are written 0800 or 08:00 or 08.00 ('O eight hundred') for 8am, 1000 or 10:00 or 10.00 for 10am, and so on.

After 12 noon you count on, so one o'clock in the afternoon, or 1pm, is 1300 hours ('thirteen hundred hours'), and so on.

Minutes after the hour are written as follows: twenty minutes past three is 1520 or 15:20 or 15.20 – 'fifteen twenty'; 5 past ten in the evening is 2205 or 22:05 or 22.05 – 'twenty-two oh five'; 6.45pm is 1845 or 18:45 or 18.45 – 'eighteen forty-five'.

The best way to become familiar with the 24-hour clock is to use it. Don't avoid the 24-hour times when you come across them; give yourself a moment to reflect.

 Activities – Working with time

Think about these questions and note down the answers in your maths diary.

Task 1

In what contexts do you come across the 24-hour clock?

Task 2

What would help you to remember the '24-hour' times? Perhaps you regularly travel by train, or work shifts which are denoted in 24-hour times.

Task 3

Convert these times to 24-hour times:

6.50pm is _____
9.15am is _____

Task 4

Convert these times to a.m./p.m. hour times:

1935 is _____
20:45 is _____

▶ 3.8   Conversions

Weight
You need to have a working knowledge of conversions from UK imperial to SI units in order to communicate with patients; you *don't* generally need to calculate conversions exactly. It may be useful to know, for example, that an adult of 63.5kg weighs 10 stone, while an infant weighing 4.54kg weighs 10 pounds (10lb), as shown in Table 5.

Table 5   *Metric conversion – weight*

Kilograms (kg)	Pounds (lb)	Ounces (oz)	Kilograms (kg)	Stones (st)	Pounds (lb)
1.36	3	0	19.05	3	0
1.47	3	4	20.87	3	4
1.59	3	8	22.23	3	7
1.70	3	12	24.04	3	11
1.81	4	0	25.40	4	0
1.93	4	4	27.22	4	4
2.04	4	8	28.58	4	7
2.15	4	12	30.39	4	11
2.27	5	0	31.75	5	0
2.38	5	4	33.57	5	4
2.50	5	8	34.93	5	7
2.61	5	12	36.74	5	11
2.72	6	0	38.10	6	0
2.84	6	4	39.92	6	4
2.95	6	8	41.28	6	7
3.06	6	12	43.09	6	11
3.18	7	0	44.45	7	0
3.29	7	4	46.27	7	4
3.40	7	8	47.63	7	7
3.52	7	12	49.44	7	11
3.63	8	0	50.88	8	0
3.74	8	4	52.62	8	4
3.86	8	8	53.98	8	7
3.97	8	12	55.79	8	11
4.08	9	0	57.15	9	0
4.20	9	4	58.97	9	4
4.31	9	8	60.33	9	7
4.42	9	12	62.14	9	11
4.54	10	0	63.50	10	0

Height

Again, you don't have to convert accurately between metres and feet and inches but it's useful to have a sense of the relationship between the two systems of measurement.

For example, a woman of medium height would be around 1.65m, or 5 feet 5 inches tall, as shown in Table 6.

Table 6   *Metric conversion – height*

Metres (m)	Feet (ft)	Inches (ins)
1.22	4	0
1.25	4	1
1.27	4	2
1.30	4	3
1.32	4	4
1.35	4	5
1.37	4	6
1.40	4	7
1.42	4	8
1.45	4	9
1.47	4	10
1.50	4	11
1.52	5	0
1.55	5	1
1.58	5	2
1.60	5	3
1.63	5	4
1.65	5	5
1.68	5	6
1.70	5	7
1.73	5	8
1.75	5	9
1.78	5	10
1.80	5	11
1.83	6	0

Temperature

In the Celsius (or Centigrade) scale the freezing point of water is 0°C and the boiling point of water is 100°C; normal body temperature is around 37°C. The Celsius scale replaces the Fahrenheit scale, which has 32°F as the freezing point and 212°F as the boiling point of water, giving a normal body temperature of around 98.6°F.

To convert °Fahrenheit to °Celsius
Take 32 away from the number of Fahrenheit degrees, multiply the result by 5 and then divide by 9 to get your answer in °C.

For example, to convert 212°F to °C, say:
212 − 32 = 180
180 × 5 = 900
900 ÷ 9 = 100°C

To convert °Celsius to °Fahrenheit
Multiply the number of degrees Celsius by 9, then divide by 5; finally add 32 to the result to get your answer in °F.

For example, to convert 20°C to °F, say:
20 × 9 = 180
180 ÷ 5 = 36
36 + 32 = 68°F

Food energy values
If you need to convert from kilocalories to kilojoules, remember that 1 kilocalorie = 4.187 kilojoules.

This means that you multiply the number of kilocalories by 4.187 to find the number of kilojoules.

If you need to convert from kilojoules to kilocalories, remember that 1 kilojoule = 0.239 kilocalorie.

Multiply the number of kilojoules by 0.239 to find the number of kilocalories.

Answers

▶ Part one   Learning and you

1.2   Developing learning strategies and study skills

Task 1   Which number-crunching method do you prefer?

1 It will take the man between 5 to14 weeks to reach a target weight in the range 58–83kg.

2 The baby's weight goes down to 3 600g (3.6kg) during the first two weeks.

3. The dose in millilitres is $\frac{62.5}{25}$ = 2.5ml.

4 0.075mg = 75 micrograms.

Task 4   Developing a feel for what's likely

Injecting an adult with 50ml of digoxin is likely when very rapid control is needed.

Giving a patient 50ml of medicine orally is unlikely.

A prescription of phenobarbitone 180mg orally at night is within the normal range for an adult.

Giving 0.02ml as an oral dose is unlikely.

An application of ichthammol ointment 3 times daily is likely.

Giving a child 6 tablets in one dose is unlikely.

▶ Part two   Calculations in the healthcare context

2.1   Monitoring vital signs

Task 1

A patient with hypothermia would have a temperature below 35°C.

Task 2

The patient's pulse pressure is 50mmHg.

Task 3
The patient's temperature has risen by 3°C overnight. This is a significant rise because she has become hyperpyrexic (i.e. with a body temperature above 39°C).

Task 4
The woman's respiration rate is almost twice the normal rate.

Task 5
The man's pulse is 15–35 beats per minute below the average normal pulse rate.

2.2   Measuring weight and height
Task 3
It will take her 5–10 weeks to reach her target weight.

Task 4
The boy was underweight.

Task 5
13.59kg is 13 kilograms and 59 grams. The patient weighs 14kg to the nearest kilogram.

Task 6
The child should be given 500mg in each dose.

2.3   The fluid balance chart
Task 1
Ms Green's total intravenous fluid intake in the period from 0800 hours to midnight is 1 500ml.

Task 2
Ms Green has taken 630ml of fluid orally.

Task 3
Ms Green has passed 650ml of urine.

Task 4
Ms Green's total fluid intake is 2 130ml; her total fluid output is 650ml.

2.4 Nutrition

Task 3

Two small slices of wholemeal bread (250kJ × 2) with butter (150kJ × 2) and jam (60kJ × 2) and a cup of tea without sugar (80kJ): total approximately 1000kJ.

Rice (150kJ) with grilled chicken (580kJ) and lettuce (40kJ): total approximately 770kJ.

Task 4

1 The patient's BMI is 22.
2 The patient's BMI is 27.5.
3 The patient's BMI is 39.
4 The patient's BMI is 17.
5 The patient's BMI is 21.
6 The patient's BMI is 23.
7 The patient's BMI is 29.

2.5 Infant feeding

Task 1

The baby's weight loss of 0.2kg is within the acceptable range. The normal weight loss for a baby of 3kg birth weight would be up to 0.3kg.

Task 2

The baby's weight should be 4 700g or 4.7kg.

Task 3

A weight loss of 0.6kg (2.5 – 1.9 = 0.6kg) by the end of the first week of life would give you cause for concern in this case because the baby has lost more than 10% of his birth weight – in fact he's lost 24% of his birth weight.

You can work this out as: $0.6 \div 2.5 \times 100 = 24\%$; or as $\frac{0.6}{2.5} \times 100 = 24\%$.

Task 4

The total fluid and energy required per day for a 10-week-old baby weighing 5kg is: 1 000ml fluid; 2 700kJ energy.

Task 5

A baby weighing 6kg should be given 200ml of fluid and 540kJ of energy in each feed if she is fed 6 times a day.

Task 6
A baby weighing 3kg should be given 100ml fluid and 270kJ energy in each feed if he is fed at 4-hourly intervals.

2.6   Giving medication
Task 1
You need two 5ml teaspoonsful for each dose.

Task 2
You need three aspirin 300mg tablets for a dose of 900mg.

Task 3
You need three tablets with 500mg in each.

Task 4   Recognition
In Simple Linctus BP citric acid monohydrate is listed by weight; all the other ingredients are listed by volume.

Task 5   Calculation
A patient on this dose would take 15 to 20ml in a day.

Task 6   Metric measurement
(a)   The main constituent of the linctus by volume is syrup.
(b)   In descending order by volume: chloroform spirit 0.3ml; amaranth solution 0.075ml; concentrated anise water 0.05ml.

Task 7
The woman should be given 3 tablets at each dose.

Task 8
3 tablets of risperidone are needed.

Task 9
You would give 11ml to the patient.

Task 10
You should give 2 suppositories.

Task 11
6 vials would be required for a dose of 200mg 3 times in 24 hours.

Task 12

A drug given in 2% solution means that the active element is 2 parts in every hundred, i.e. 2 grams of the active element in 100ml or 2 000mg in every 100ml or 20mg in every 1ml (20mg/ml).

Task 13

The infusion rate works out exactly as 16.6 drops per millilitre but this is not practicable; to the nearest drop it is 17 drops per millilitre.

Task 14

The infusion rate is 125 drops per millilitre.

2.7 Staffing and budget calculations

Task 1

£19 000 income per week is generated when the home is full.

Task 2

The costs rise by £1 176.

Task 3

(a)   You would make £300 000 profit.
(b)   Profits are 30% of income.

Task 4

The Whole Time Equivalents of a clerical officer, assuming 1 clerical WTE = 35 hours per week, are:

17.5 hours = 0.5 WTE
0.75 WTE = 26.25 hours (i.e. 26 hours 15 minutes)
14 hours = 0.4 WTE
0.25 WTE = 8.75 hours (i.e. 8 hours 45 minutes)

Task 5

The nursing hours and WTEs, assuming 1 nursing WTE is 37.5 hours, are:

0.5 WTE = 18.75 hours (i.e. 18 hours 45 minutes) per week
0.75 WTE = 28.125 hours (i.e. 28 hours 7.5 minutes) per week
12 hours per week = 0.32 WTE
9 hours per week = 0.24 WTE

Task 6
The annual leave entitlements are:

1 21
2 22.5
3 13
4 11
5 23

2.8 Demographic profiles
Task 3
Approximately 14% of the population of the Borough of Lewisham is over 65; approximately 16% are pensioners.

Task 4
(a) 28 377 pensioners in Lewisham live alone.
(b) This is approximately 37% of the total number of pensioners in Lewisham.

▶ Part three   Maths refreshers

3.1   Whole numbers
Task 1
In the number 527, the 2 means 20.

Task 2
In the number 72 543, the 2 means 2,000.

Task 3
63 987 is sixty-three thousand, nine hundred and eighty-seven.

Task 4
260 001 is two hundred and sixty thousand and one; 8 007 639 is eight million, seven thousand, six hundred and thirty-nine; 39 124 228 is thirty-nine million, one hundred and twenty-four thousand, two hundred and twenty-eight.

3.2   The 'four rules' of arithmetic
Task 1
Whichever way you add the numbers, the total is 5 629.

Task 2
$360 \div 9 = 40$

Task 3
$48 \times 100 = 4\,800$

Task 4
$6(4\,789 - 650) = 24\,834$

Task 5
$(76 + 450) - (240 \div 8) = 496$

Task 6
7 830 is 7.830×10^3 expressed in standard form.

Task 7
10^{-5} expressed as a decimal is 0.000 01.

Task 8
Here are the numbers arranged in size order with the largest number first:
4^8; 4^6; 4^3; 4^2.

3.4 Decimals and fractions
Task 1
$0.01 = \frac{1}{100}$

Task 2
$\frac{7}{20} = 0.35$

Task 3
$0.25 \times 3.64 = 0.91$

Task 4
$\frac{42.5}{25} = 1.7$

Task 5
$0.008\,1 \div 0.9 = 0.009$

Task 6
$\frac{75}{100} + \frac{20}{80} = 1$

Task 7

$\frac{16}{32} = \frac{1}{2}$; $\frac{50}{200} = \frac{1}{4}$; $\frac{25}{150} = \frac{1}{6}$; $\frac{36}{540} = \frac{1}{15}$

3.4   Percentages

Task 1

50% of 600 = 300

15% of 4 500 = 675

Task 2

3 litres of 10% dextrose contain 0.3 litres of dextrose

(i.e. $\frac{10}{100} \times 3L = 0.3L$)

Task 3

500 is 2% of 25 000; 200 is 2.5% of 8 000

Task 4

3 000 people are likely to have heart disease.

3.5   Ratios

Task 2

5:100 = 1:20; 6:12 = 1:2; 25:50 = 1:2

Task 3

25:100 = 1:4 = 2:8 = 5:20

Task 4

There is 100ml of stock solution in 600ml of diluted solution if the strength of the solution is 1:5.

3.6   The metric (SI) system

Task 1

3g = 3000mg

Task 2

600ml = 0.6L

Task 3

400ml = 0.4L

0.5g = 500mg

0.1L = 100ml
8 000mg = 8g

Task 4
59mg is 59 milligrams
74mmol/L is 74 millimoles per litre
3Mg is 3 Megagrams
4mJ is 4 millijoules

Task 5
1 000ml is the same as 1L
35g is bigger than 35mg
200L is bigger than 2ml

3.7   The 24-hour clock
Task 3
6.50pm is 1850
9.15am is 0915

Task 4
1935 is 7.35pm
20:45 is 8.45pm

Bibliography

Adair, J. (1988) *Effective Time Management: How To Save Time And Spend It Wisely*. London: Pan Books.

Bailey, D. (1994) *The NHS Budget-Holder's Survival Guide*. Harlow: Longman.

BAPEN (2004) The Malnutrition Universal Screening Tool (MUST) [online], pdf at: http://www.bapen.org.uk

BHS (2005) *Blood Pressure Management*. London: British Hypertension Society.

Bliss-Holtz, J. (1994). 'Discriminating types of medication calculation errors in nursing practice', *Nursing Research* 43(6), 373–5.

British Medical Association & Royal Pharmaceutical Society of Great Britain (2004) *British National Formulary* (biannual). London: British Medical Association and the Pharmaceutical Press (see http://bnf.org/bnf/extra/current/noframes/450016.htm).

Buxton, L. (1981) *Do You Panic About Maths? Coping with maths anxiety*. London: Heinemann Educational.

Cartwright, M. (1996). 'Numeracy needs of the beginning Registered Nurse', *Nurse Education Today* 16, 137–43.

Cernik, K. & Wearne, M. (1992) 'Using community health profiles to improve service provision', *Health Visitor* 65(10), 343–5.

Coben, D. & Atere-Roberts, E. (1996). *Carefree Calculations for Healthcare Students*. Basingstoke, Macmillan.

Coben, D. & Black, S. (2005) *The Numeracy Pack* (4th edn). London: Basic Skills Agency.

Coben, D. & Thumpston, G. (1996) 'Common sense, good sense and invisible mathematics', in T. Kjærgård, A. Kvamme and N. Lindén (eds), *PDME III Proceedings: Numeracy, Gender, Class, Race*, Proceedings of the Third International Conference of Political Dimensions of Mathematics Education (PDME) III, Bergen, Norway, 24–27 July 1995. Landås, Norway: Caspar, 284–98.

Dexter, M. & Applegate, P. (1990) 'How to solve a math problem', *Journal of Nursing Education* 9(2), 49–53.

Fulton, W. H. & O'Neill, G. P. (1989) 'Mathematics anxiety

drug dose calculation', *Journal of Nursing Education* 28(8), October, 343–6.

Hek, G. (1994) 'Adding up the cost of teaching mathematics', *Nursing Standard* 8(22), 23 February, 25–9.

Hoyles, C., Noss, R. & Pozzi, S. (1999) 'Mathematising in practice', in C. Hoyles, C. Morgan & G. Woodhouse (eds), *Rethinking the Mathematics Curriculum*. London: Falmer, 48–62.

Hoyles, C., Noss, R. & Pozzi, S. (2001) 'Proportional reasoning in nursing practice', *Journal for Research in Mathematics Education* 32(1), 4–27.

Hutton, B. M. (1998a) 'Student nurses and mathematics' in D. Coben & J. O'Donoghue (eds), *Adults Learning Maths-4: Proceedings of ALM-4, the Fourth International Conference of Adults Learning Maths – A Research Forum held at University of Limerick, Ireland, July 4-6 1997*. London: Goldsmith's College, University of London in association with ALM, 192–8.

Hutton, B. M. (1998b) 'Should nurses carry calculators?', in D. Coben & J. O'Donoghue (eds), *Adults Learning Maths-4: Proceedings of ALM-4, the Fourth International Conference of Adults Learning Maths – A Research Forum held at University of Limerick, Ireland, July 4-6 1997*. London: Goldsmith's College, University of London in association with ALM, 164–72.

Hutton, B. M. (2000). 'Numeracy must become a priority for nurses', *British Journal of Nursing* 9(14), 894.

Insley, J. (1996) *A Paediatric Vade-Mecum* (13th edn). London: Arnold.

Lave, J. & Wenger, E. (1991) *Situated Learning: Legitimate peripheral participation*. Cambridge: Cambridge University Press.

Miller, J. (1993) 'Solving the problem', *Nursing Times* 89(43), 40–1.

Noss, R., Hoyles, C. & Pozzi, S. (1998) Towards a mathematical orientation through computational modeling. ESRC end of award report. London: Mathematical Sciences Group, Institute of Education, University of London.

Pirie   (1981) *Mathematics in Medicine. A report for the Cockcroft* ` Shell Centre, University of Nottingham.

'Deficiencies in basic mathematical skills among nurses: `d evaluation of methods of detection and treatment'. `ity of Nottingham.

`d Mathematics: Deficiencies in Basic Mathematical `on: Royal College of Nursing.

` in Practice-Based Calculation: Issues for `ew of the literature. London: Learning and Teaching Support Network (LTSN) Centre for Health Sciences and Practice.

Schoenfeld, A. (1994). Reflections on doing and teaching mathematics. In A. Schoenfeld (ed.), *Mathematical Thinking and Problem Solving*. Hillsdale, NJ: Lawrence Erlbaum, 53-69.

Shockley, J. S., McGurn, W. C., Gunning, C., Graveley, E. & Tillotson, D. (1989) 'Effects of calculator use on arithmetic and conceptual skills of nursing students', *Journal of Nursing Education* 28(9), 402-5.

Taylor, N. (1992) *Budgeting Skills: A Guide for Nurse Managers*. Lancaster: Quay Publishing.

Zaslavsky, C. (1994) *Fear of Math and How to Get Over It and Get On With Your Life!* New Brunswick, NJ: Rutgers University Press.

Index